Sleep Talking

SCIENCE, NEEDS & MISCONCEPTIONS

Yvonne Harrison

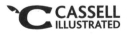
CASSELL
ILLUSTRATED

First published in the UK 1999 by Blandford
Reprinted in 2005 by Cassell Illustrated
a division of Octopus Publishing Group Limited
2-4 Heron Quays
London E14 4JP

Distributed in the United States
by Sterling Publishing Co., In c.
387 Park Avenue South, New York, NY 10016-8810

A Cataloguing-in-Publication Data entry for this title is available
and may be obtained from the British Library

ISBN 0-7137-2748-9
EAN 9780713727487

Printed and bound in Great Britain by
Mackays of Chatham plc, Chatham, Kent

Contents

Introduction

Sleep is a biological process which most of us indulge in on the assumption of some sort of renewal or revitalization. It reduces us, in a very dramatic way, to a state which has little in common with our waking life. We do not respond to the things around us, have rational thoughts or make deliberate actions. Instead, hours flash by in an instant, leaving us with only a vague, often chaotic, recollection of dream images. During sleep, we are deprived of everything that is familiar and predictable in the outside world.

For some time now there has been a growing interest in understanding the necessity for sleep: how we achieve it, how we avoid it, why we do it. The reasons for this are partly due to changes in the way we live. Until fairly recently there was only a limited number of things that could be done at night – hence sleep, in the absence of anything more exciting, was usually given a high priority. This is not the case any more: we have supermarkets, banking, business, electronic retailing, travel and communications throughout the world all available on a 24-hour basis. Many people, especially those in industrial, caring and emergency occupations, can now expect to work at all hours of the day and night. As the traditional distinction between day and night becomes more obscure, we are faced with a considerable amount of competition for our attention during a time when we would normally expect to be asleep. This is a book about how we have come to understand the role of sleep in the modern world.

Judging by the enthusiasm for radio and television programmes, newspaper and magazine articles, and books on the subject, sleep is considered to be an appropriate concern for late twentieth-century western societies. My own interest in sleep began as an undergraduate, when it became clear to me that, despite its appearing to have an obvious role, the scientific understanding of the reasons for sleep is still far from complete. Before too long I realized that we are in fact much closer to understanding *how* we sleep (when, where, for how long, etc) than *why*.

In this book, I have tried to take a step back from the idea of sleep as a purely biological process. I believe that an understanding of the significance of sleep for the body and for health is only half the story, and that the fascination extends beyond our ability to explore sleep in these terms.

How to use the book

The book is divided into four sections. Part 1 asks the question: 'What is it that is so interesting about sleep?'. Over the centuries, sleep has inspired many different religious, spiritual, magical and cultural beliefs, and has only recently being accepted as a legitimate area of scientific study.

We begin by tracing the development of a scientific interest in sleep over the last 100 years or so. Many of the early scientific researchers in this area were keen to explore the limits of animal and human endurance without sleep. It was assumed that by depriving the body of whatever process was taking place during sleep, its role (and therefore its true nature) would eventually be revealed through the emerging physical and intellectual impairments. Scientists were also aware of the complex relationship between a body's need for sleep and the influence of the environment: how far the internal 'body clock' (which reminds us of a physical need for sleep) is affected by the conditions in which we live.

This problem was addressed through a series of unusual experiments designed to separate an innate drive for sleep from the influence of environmental factors. For weeks on end, volunteers would be deprived of all natural light, exposure to the outside world or knowledge of time, leaving them with nothing more than their internal 'body clock' to rely on. Nowadays, these experiments take place in custom-built, soundproofed, windowless laboratories, but in the 1930s and 1940s scientists resorted to lengthy stays in underground caves in order to achieve the necessary level of isolation.

Through these techniques, they were able to demonstrate the human being's reliance on normal daily fluctuations in light, noise, temperature and social activity in order to 'fine tune' an internal drive to sleep. Consequently, we are not good at coping with extreme environments in which these external behavioural 'cues' are missing. These experiments have also helped towards an understanding of many of the problems experienced by shift-workers, who are regularly expected to remain awake at a time when their body is preparing for sleep.

Similar difficulties are experienced during extended space travel, where an astronaut's 'day' can be severely disrupted. Under these conditions, the body can easily be 'out of step' with the immediate environment, resulting in fatigue and mood-related problems which may compromise the overall effectiveness of the mission. It has been possible to simulate many of these difficulties through long stays in Arctic conditions, for example, and so prepare astronauts for the task ahead. The challenge, for the not-too-distant future, will be to prepare for a manned flight to Mars. For this, it will be necessary to develop novel solutions to the problems of maintaining a normal sleep/wake cycle throughout a dramatic reduction in social and behavioural stimulation. For example, how will astronauts cope with a lengthy (at least nine-month) outward journey and a Martian 'day' which lasts 37 minutes longer than the one we are used to?

Scientists are not the only group with an interest in sleep. The fascination is also shared at a popular level, with many of the earlier sleep-loss 'marathons' broadcast as media events. While the dance marathons of the 1930s and 1940s are no longer in vogue, the modern alternatives, such as the ultra-marathon (endurance running) or cine-marathon (continuous film-viewing) still demand a considerable level of sleep loss.

In this section, we also discuss the reluctance to view sleep from a purely rational and scientific perspective. It is interesting that many beliefs concerning the magical or spiritual qualities of sleep (which are reminiscent of a pre-scientific culture) are still an important feature of popular books and films.

Part 1 concludes by looking at the modern sleep laboratory and what we know about the basic sleep process. We also examine the issues currently under investigation, and the challenges for the sleep laboratory of the future.

It is difficult not to have an opinion about sleep, even if it is only in relation to your own sleep needs. Whether you are a light sleeper, a heavy sleeper, a long sleeper, a short sleeper, a morning person, a night owl, a sleep-walker, a snorer, a teeth grinder, a sleep talker, a cat napper, or a power napper, the way that you sleep says something very definite about the type of person you are. In Part 2 we take a look at some of the myths and half-truths about sleep which are currently in circulation. This section deals with some basic issues – such as how much people sleep each night, whether this changes as we get older, how to measure sleep throughout the night, etc – before going on to look at popular beliefs about sleep. We ask whether these are always consistent with the available scientific knowledge. Where do these ideas (such as the 'standard' eight hours' sleep) originate? Can common sense tell us everything we need to know about sleep? Why shouldn't we aim to sleep for six hours, or for ten? Why is it considered good to get by on very little sleep? Is society really anti-sleep? Is sleep a waste of time? Can we decide how much we sleep? Are sleep habits determined by genes or temperament? What about 'beauty' sleep, or sleep for kids? Does everybody sleep?

In Part 3, we explore the link between sleep and the inner workings of the mind. Sleep, particularly dreaming, is popularly understood to be essential for a healthy, stable frame of mind. It has been argued that the process of dreaming provides access to the complexities of the troubled mind and the means of restoring spiritual and psychological harmony. If this is the case, then you would predict severe psychological trauma if a person were deprived of the opportunity to dream, but to date there is no convincing evidence for this.

So why the obsession with dreaming? In recent years, we have witnessed the emergence of a large industry of 'dream-workers' in response to a need to know and, importantly, a willingness to talk about our dreams. We explore the notion that this reflects a more general preoccupation with the process of self-disclosure as a route to self-knowledge, and ask whether the scientific study of dreaming has been exhausted.

This section also includes a discussion of our willingness to invest sleep with phenomena which are not easily explained in scientific terms. These include claims to precognitive experiences – such as premonitions of personal and public events, and travel outside the body during sleep. Again, there is no convincing scientific evidence for these phenomena. So why do we expect so much from our dreams?

In the final section, we look at what might be considered to be more 'applied' issues concerning sleep and the demands of a modern world. What is there left to know about sleep? The scientific study of sleep began in earnest approximately 100 years ago. There have been a number of triumphs along the way, in particular the detection of distinct and universal patterns of brain activity during sleep. However, despite the more sophisticated techniques of modern sleep research, many of the questions raised by the first researchers remain unanswered: the very basic one of why we sleep springs to mind.

What is particularly interesting, though, is the way in which scientific research has been able to respond to changes in our daily activity patterns over recent years – issues such as falling asleep while driving a car or operating dangerous machinery, and coping with the demands of working through the night or for prolonged periods without sleep. How do we make decisions in critical situations when we are desperate for sleep?

We have also seen the emergence of contemporary legal issues involving sleep, to which the modern sleep researcher has been invited to contribute. These debates look at questions such as whether we have a duty to sleep, if by not sleeping we endanger ourselves or others, and whether or not we are responsible for our actions during sleep. There are many reports of individuals making cups of tea, negotiating dangerous stairways or even driving a car while sound asleep, but although the majority of these events are harmless, from time to time the consequences of actions during sleep can have devastating effects.

In February 1961 a 29-year-old US Air Force sergeant based in Essex, England, was acquitted of the murder of a young woman after convincing the court that he had been asleep as he strangled her to death. The judge presumed this to be a most unusual defence: 'Have you ever heard of a man strangling a woman while he was asleep? Does there exist any record that such things happen?' In fact, there are many records of similar cases throughout the world, and this was by no means the first time the courts had been asked to decide on responsibility for actions which take place during sleep. If it can be shown that the defendant was not aware of the attack as it took place, and had no control over it, then it is quite likely that a 'not guilty' verdict will be reached.

Then what about 'lucid dreaming'? This is a relatively new but extremely popular technique aimed at enhancing the dream experience. It is claimed that we all have the potential to make radical changes to the way that we dream, and that, with training, we can eventually expect to control many of the features, including the storylines, characters and locations. So, does knowing that we are dreaming as it happens, and being able to control the outcome, put us under a legal obligation to behave ourselves during sleep?

Many of the current issues have emerged as a result of a concern for the way we live our lives. In this 24-hour society, are we really too busy to fulfil our basic need for sleep – and if so, what can be done to resolve this conflict? Finally, we ask whether there will ever be a point when we can do without sleep and whether we are near to providing a substitute for our dependence on the idea of the standard eight hours' each night.

The title *Sleep Talking* is intended to reflect the ongoing discussions about sleep which are current across a range of social agencies: scientific, medical, legislative, judicial, educational and social. A limited amount of necessary scientific detail concerning the 'mechanics' of the sleep process is included in the early chapters. From this point on, it is intended that each chapter will be self-contained, and you should be able to 'dip' into any particular issue and explore the fascinating world of sleep from whatever perspective captures your interest.

Part 1

A fascination with sleep

Chapter 1
A scientific quest

What is it that is so fascinating about sleep? Whether we grudgingly give in to sleep, or succumb with relish, most people plan to do it at least once in every 24-hour period. We expect to feel better for it, but that is not always the case. We are concerned when things go wrong, and are quick to look for an explanation in terms of our waking life. Whether it is through the stress of overwork, illness or relationships, lack of sleep is often seen as a useful 'barometer' of our overall state of well-being – so much so that sleep is thought to be intricately linked with almost every area of our lives. From work through to pleasure, getting a good night's sleep can make all the difference between being efficient or forgetful, lethargic or full of energy, irritable or easy-going.

This chapter focuses on attempts to understand sleep from a scientific point of view, beginning with a discussion of the early experimental approach and the types of questions which were to establish sleep as both an interesting and legitimate area of scientific research. Experiments in isolation units suggested that we have a powerful internal body 'clock' which keeps time with remarkable accuracy even when the environment is completely stripped of all artificial time cues. We are essentially creatures of habit, with 'good' and 'bad' times to sleep, and yet we are also essentially social in nature, and live in a technologically sophisticated world in which the original divisions between day and night no longer hold true. These experiments generated fundamental questions concerning sleep, many of which are still relevant today. Why do we sleep? How do we know when to sleep? How far are we free to choose when to sleep?

Understanding sleep

Sleep has been identified as a major 'human factor' problem for the twenty-first century. The convenience, or necessity, of a 24-hour society has meant that we now spend more time awake when the body is expecting to be asleep than ever before. Clearly, it is no longer desirable for us all to be asleep at the same time. In a bid to achieve patterns of sleep and wake 'on demand', we are forced to rely heavily on artificial aids, such as sleeping pills and caffeine.

However, there is some concern that we have now moved so far away from our natural rhythm of sleep, that we have forgotten what it feels like to be wide awake without such aids.

The modern 'scientific' study of sleep is often said to have emerged about 100 years ago, beginning with a series of experiments designed to test the limits of human endurance without sleep. This was a time of great enthusiasm for the systematic investigation of all areas of human life. Sleep was a natural focus, because of the assumption that regular sleep was essential for achieving the 'best' from our abilities. Industrialization in western countries was also gathering momentum and the universities were starting to make a concerted effort towards understanding the 'human' contribution to this process. This coincided with a shift in work demands towards large-scale production processes centred around repetitive, monotonous and drawn-out tasks, which in turn introduced concerns for fatigue, efficiency, safety and productivity. All these issues are indirectly related to the need for sleep.

The enthusiasm for the scientific study of sleep has been fuelled over the years by a number of landmark, occasionally fortuitous, discoveries and, perhaps above all, a willingness to respond to the problems thrown up by an increasingly complex society.

There have been a number of important technological developments which have helped to advance the study of sleep. In particular, the development of the electroencephalogram (EEG) in the 1930s led to the discovery of a distinct and universal pattern of brain activity during sleep. We know more about the qualitative aspects of sleep than ever before. We also know a lot about 'normal' sleep and how the body responds to changes in the immediate environment.

Today, there are two fundamental questions that continue to frustrate and intrigue scientists:
• What are the reasons for sleep?
• Why do we sleep when we do?

Who needs sleep?

Over the years sleep has been credited with many functions, some of which are more convincing than others. For example, it could be a time for organizing the experiences of the day – a sort of mental 'housekeeping', clearing out the clutter of unnecessary information and filing away only the essential memories for future reference and easy access. Perhaps we need sleep to grow, so that it is particularly important for children, or for sorting through emotional worries. Is it perhaps a rest for the brain, or simply a means of keeping us safe during the hours of darkness?

The idea that we can understand the reasons for sleep by observing the effects of not sleeping has an intuitive appeal. Many experiments have been designed around this premise, only to find – to the frustration of those involved – that there are no straightforward or simple answers to unravelling the mystery of why we sleep. In the early years, scientists were willing to go to great lengths in pursuit of this goal. Acting as both experimenters and volunteers, they would often deprive themselves and fellow volunteers of three to four nights without sleep. During these experiments, systematic recordings would be made of physical or psychological functioning for which some effect of sleep loss was anticipated; these included heart rate, respiration, mood, reaction time, cognition, visual or auditory hallucinations and so on.

At this stage there was every reason to think that staying awake for long periods was a risky proposition, as the only precedent to these experiments involved animals, who invariably died when the periods of sleep loss were taken to an extreme. Fortunately, this was not the case in experiments with humans – but then they did have the advantage of being able to withdraw from the experiment at any time. In fact, very few serious effects have ever been reported, and at worse these are completely reversed after sleep is resumed.

However, it became clear quite early on, following the publication of a disparate and often conflicting range of accounts, that one of the most important factors governing a response to prolonged periods of sleep deprivation was individual tolerance. While some people complained of dizziness, headaches, extreme fatigue, visual hallucinations and double vision towards the end of a lengthy experiment without sleep, others had relatively little difficulty at all. It was perhaps surprising to learn just how much we are capable of without sleep. For example, an experiment at the University of Chicago in the 1920s found that students performed just as well in a difficult examination whether they had slept the night before or not[1]. Their results were pretty much indistinguishable following either a good night's sleep or after having stayed up all night as part of the experiment, although the students felt that they had to try that bit harder to stay attentive because of their tiredness. This may be encouraging for today's students who plan their own revision timetable around sleepless nights, but it is probably not something to be relied on, bearing in mind the more subtle changes in mood following a night without sleep, which are likely to have some additional impact on exam performance.

Over the years a number of individuals have been so convinced that they can manage completely without sleep that they have volunteered themselves for 'open-ended' sleep deprivation studies. In 1933, for example, a young man, referred to in subsequent reports as Z, came forward with the suggestion that he could go without sleep indefinitely and was prepared to do so under experimental conditions. The result was a remarkable 231 hours (almost ten full days) without sleep before Z finally decided that he had had enough.

However, the longest recorded period of sleep loss in humans did not take place inside a laboratory, but instead was initiated as part of a public sleep-loss 'marathon'. The media picked up on this idea in the 1960s, when on separate occasions three young, healthy American men set out to destroy the myth of sleep. The first attempt was made by a young radio disc jockey by the name of Peter Tripp, who managed to stay awake for around 200 hours. Throughout this time he was stationed in a broadcasting booth in the middle of Times Square, New York, and made the most of his short-lived celebrity status by raising money for a national child-care charity, the March of Dimes. This was followed shortly afterwards by another young disc jockey, John Hart, managing to stay awake for 252 hours (over ten days) and continuing broadcasting his regular radio programme throughout – an almost unimaginable feat for most people. Both emotionally and psychologically, Hart apparently coped well with his experience. At the low points he described minor visual hallucinations and a sense of disorientation, but he bounced back to his normal self fairly quickly after finally succumbing to sleep.

Unfortunately for Hart, he was soon to be relieved of his 'record' by a 17-year-old by the name of Randy Gardner. Based in San Diego, he stayed awake for a total of 264 hours, an incredible 11 days and nights. After attracting the attention of a local radio station, it became clear within a few days that this was no ordinary stunt. Medics and researchers from a nearby university volunteered themselves to monitor Gardner's well-being and to confirm that he was in fact awake throughout. His achievement has since been quoted widely in the scientific and popular literature, perhaps because, quite apart from anything else, he seemed to defy all common sense by being able to go without sleep for so long. First-hand descriptions of Gardner's mood and demeanour throughout the 11 nights suggest that he had very few problems, and those he did experience were centred mainly around memory and speech, but none was serious. Interestingly, when he finally went to sleep, he had only one or two nights of longer-than-normal sleep before feeling fully recovered.

It is not clear whether everybody would cope quite so well for so long without sleep, and surely very few would be willing even to try. Tripp, Hart and Gardner were all young, healthy, well prepared mentally, and probably enjoyed the attention they were attracting, and these factors are likely to have been important in their success. Despite the difficulties endured towards the end, none of them is reported to have suffered long-term effects from his extended period without sleep. Given their original ideals, it is difficult to know whether in fact these young men were compelled by a need to sleep by day ten or eleven and could not face going on, or whether they simply realized the futility of their quest beyond their original record-breaking aims. It seems likely that many more 'marathons' of this kind took place without attracting media attention, and some may even be planned (although, as we shall see, there are a number of reasons why this should be discouraged).

One of the problems with all psychological studies, including sleep-loss experiments, is that volunteers bring their own expectations to the undertaking. This had a positive effect for Peter Tripp, John Hart and Randy Gardner who, because of their strength of will and determination, were able to adopt an extremely positive attitude and were enthusiastic about going without sleep. Their complaints seem to have been on a par with, or even more minor than, those of volunteers who have taken part in experiments involving far shorter periods without sleep.

The importance of mental preparedness may explain why there is such an obvious difference between the outcome of extremely long-term studies of sleep deprivation and the more general assumption that prolonged periods without sleep are harmful. Under normal circumstances it is not only extremely rare to go without sleep for so long but, should the need arise, it is nearly always under severe, perhaps hostile, conditions. It is well known that the effects of sleep loss are compounded by stressful situations leading to extreme vulnerability. Since the time of the Spanish Inquisition, the idea of depriving people of sleep against their will has been seen as a powerful tool in securing confessions at all costs. More recently, the right to sleep during modern interrogation procedures is recognized by the European Human Rights Commission as a basic right of all citizens coming under its jurisdiction, and there are firm guidelines to ensure adequate provision for regular sleep in criminal investigations.

Very few scientists nowadays are engaged in researching long-term sleep deprivation, as these extremes have little bearing on most people's lives. While the early experiments were perhaps inspired by a fascination for the extreme, sleep-loss experiments nowadays are more likely to reflect the sorts of periods which are normal in everyday life, and are motivated by a need to understand individual tolerance in order, for example, to improve working conditions. One night without sleep is common for many professions, such as the medical and emergency services, with perhaps only military agencies having any interest in longer periods.

An enormous amount of data has been collected from sleep-deprivation experiments of this kind over the past few decades, and it has generated perhaps as many questions as answers. For example, we still don't know how important motivation is in overcoming the effects of sleep loss: given the vast differences in the coping strategies employed, we can only guess. There is also the difficulty of knowing just how far 'mock' situations in laboratories can give any real indication of how people will perform under more genuine circumstances, particularly when other stresses are involved, such as in life or death situations. But perhaps the most important question at the moment asks just how long a person should be allowed to continue working without sleep in the event of an emergency. The prevailing view seems to be that today's decision-maker should see a crisis through to the end, and that the responsibility of being in charge will override any serious physical or psychological impairment stemming from a need for sleep. And yet there is compelling evidence to suggest that insufficient sleep is a critical factor in many of the recent major public catastrophes (see Chapter 12).

Why do we sleep when we do?

Considering that at the turn of the century scientists had little more than observation, introspection and some relatively unrefined psychological techniques to rely on, the early experiments in sleep loss offered a quite remarkable insight into the sleep process. It was only years later that many of these findings were to be confirmed by objective means, following the development of more sophisticated tools for examining the activity of the brain during sleep.

One of the more consistent observations from these experiments was that, rather than getting progressively worse as time went by, volunteers invariably complained of feeling profoundly sleepy at one moment, only to be almost fully alert at the next. If plotted on a graph, these changes showed a distinct pattern or 'rhythm' of discomfort throughout the trials. The lowest time for most people was between 2am and 6am, and perhaps again in the early afternoon, whereas during the mid-morning period and early evening many of them were reported to be surprisingly active and free from the worst effects of sleepiness. This 'rhythm' in energy and alertness may go some way towards encouraging volunteers to persevere with the experiment, knowing even at their worst moments that things will eventually improve.

A biological 'body clock'?

These fluctuations were to alert researchers to the powerful influence of a rhythmic process, which reminds us of a body's need to alternate sleep and wakefulness on a regular basis. This pattern appears to be dominated by changes which reflect the natural distinction between day and night. The term 'circadian' (meaning 'around a day') was used to describe the daily regularity of this pattern, but where does it originate? The obvious suggestion is that we have an internal 'alarm clock' of some sort which is activated to signal that it is time to sleep. If that is the case, does it keep good time and why is this important?

The early experiments hinted at a powerful internal drive, or biological rhythm, for sleep which waxes and wanes at regular intervals throughout a 24-hour period. But it is the urge to sleep – experienced as sleepiness – rather than sleep itself which is rhythmical. The decision to respond to this urge is largely dependent on our own will to do so (with the exception of overpowering sleepiness due to illness or extreme sleep deprivation).

External factors

The relationship between this internal rhythm reminding us to sleep and a whole range of external factors is a complex one. There are many social opportunities and strategies available through which we ignore the body's 'cue' to sleep: by staying mobile, seeking out company, drinking strong coffee. There are also patterns in the environment which provide a strong reminder to sleep or to stay awake, such as daylight and darkness. So, just how important are these factors?

One way to get to grips with this question has been to examine the natural rhythms of the body in total isolation, ie with absolutely no artificial schedule on which to rely. Today's laboratory is well equipped to deal with these 'time-free' experiments as they are known, being able to provide soundproofed isolation units with constant light, and carefully controlled activity. Volunteers may be deprived of all natural light, exposure to the outside world and knowledge of time, leaving them with nothing more than their internal 'body clock' to rely on. Laboratory staff work irregular and unpredictable shifts and are trained to avoid giving away any clues as to the time of day or night. This means that volunteers have to rely solely on how they are feeling in order to decide when it is time to wake up and time to go to sleep.

Early experimenters had to resort to more extreme measures, submerging themselves and their volunteers for months on end in isolated underground chambers or caverns. Under these conditions, many unusual patterns of activity emerged. It seems that the 24-hour day is not 100 per cent consistent with the body's own rhythm, which for many people may be closer to a 24½–25-hour 'day'. The fact that on the whole we choose to follow a 24-hour day suggests a compromise between a biological or internally driven rhythm and the natural and social rhythms of the world in which we live.

Factors which regulate our decision to sleep are known as 'zeitgebers', and include all aspects of a daily routine – particularly work schedules, meal times, leisure, family, domestic commitments and social activity. We also schedule our behaviours around natural zeitgebers in the environment such as fluctuations in light, darkness and temperature. The concept of zeitgebers is an important idea in relation to understanding many of the questions concerning when and for how long we sleep, as well as many of the difficulties which have arisen from attempts to reschedule sleep/wake patterns, during shiftwork for example. In time-free experiments we observe a 'drift' away from the 24-hour day because of the reduction in available external zeitgebers. As the richness of our normal environments is reduced, we are left to rely on internal rhythms. Then as the period of isolation increases, volunteers can eventually become totally out of step with the outside world.

However, what is fascinating to observe from these experiments is that for some people the body is extremely accurate in measuring 'time' when all natural external cues (daylight) and artificial external cues (social activity) are removed. There is a remarkable tendency towards regularity despite losing step with the 24-hour day. At one extreme, for example, in the 1980s a young French pot-holer, Veronique L. Geun, spent 110 days in total isolation in a 77m (250ft) deep cave in the Causses mountains in southern France. During this time she lived to a 50-hour 'day', spending 20 hours asleep followed by 30 hours awake.

Such experiments have helped to show how important external zeitgebers are in 'fine-tuning' an internal 'clock'. For this reason, they have made an invaluable contribution towards understanding the more extreme demands of modern living. Shiftwork and regular trans-global travel force us into a situation where the physical state of the body is out of step with the world around us. This leads to conflicting messages between how we feel physically (due to the phase of the biological clock) and how the outside world expects us to feel. So just how flexible is the biological 'clock'?

Are we tied to a 24-hour day?

Throughout a series of intriguing experiments in the 1930s and 1940s, two professors from the University of Chicago, Dr Kleitman and Dr Richardson[2], demonstrated that it was possible to break away from the 24-hour day and live with some success on a different 'day' length – either slightly longer (28 hours) or slightly shorter (21 hours). This involved completely ignoring the 'earth' day (measured by a single revolution around the sun), and living instead to a strict alternative timetable of bedtimes and waketimes.

Because of the distractions of a busy laboratory which provided a constant reminder of the 24-hour pattern of life, the professors eventually resorted to trying out this experiment (on themselves) in a well known Kentucky tourist attraction – the Mammoth Caves. Their 'laboratory' was set up in an underground cave offering an environment of total natural darkness and near-constant temperature all the year round. They had also arranged for no unnecessary contact with the outside world, other than the delivery of supplies.

Throughout these experiments, Kleitman and Richardson followed a predetermined day length which was slightly different to their normal aboveground routine. This would be strictly imposed by going to bed and getting up at set times, no matter how sleepy they felt. During the 'day' periods they would remain active within the cave, reading and working (this required some dim artificial lighting), while during the designated 'night' periods they would retire to their beds and lie there in total darkness throughout, the idea being that only limited, carefully scheduled opportunities for sleep were available.

Having assumed beforehand that it might take some time for the body to adjust to these new schedules, Kleitman and Richardson prepared to spend whole months at a time in their underground laboratory. As it turned out, they found that they were able to follow these regimes and live quite success-fully on a routine of both long (28-hour) and short (21-hour) days. Note that the 'night' period, the opportunity for sleep, was maintained at around eight hours, and it was the active period or 'day' which was adjusted to accommodate either a shortened or lengthened day/night cycle.

Fig 1 illustrates how this can be achieved in relation to the 'outside' world. If you were thinking about adopting either of these routines, you can see that this means sleeping at all hours of the normal 24-hour clock, and not just between midnight and 8am as most people are used to. It also means sleeping out of synchrony with natural daylight, a factor which causes con-siderable problems for today's shiftworker. The difficulty with this lies in getting good 'quality' sleep when the time for sleep conflicts with the body's

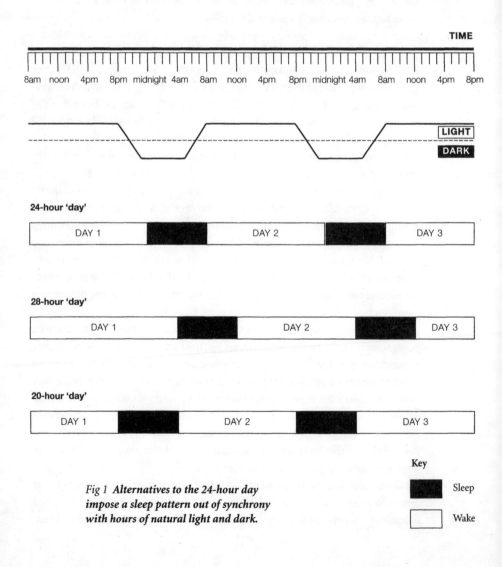

Fig 1 Alternatives to the 24-hour day impose a sleep pattern out of synchrony with hours of natural light and dark.

natural time for alertness. In underground caves, or in other isolated situations, this problem is reduced, because it is possible for the 'bedroom' to be made quiet and distractions kept to a minimum during the specified sleep periods. In the real world, of course, this is not always possible, and the noise and activity associated with certain periods of the day means that novel sleeping schedules such as these would be extremely difficult to achieve.

Nevertheless, these experiments demonstrated that under certain conditions the body is not tied to a 24-hour pattern of sleep and activity, as might be assumed, but that variations in a normal 'day' length are possible. Again, individual tolerance, particularly to the stress of isolation, is extremely important.

Natural zeitgeber reductions – the polar regions

There are an increasing number of situations for which the social and environmental zeitgebers are either weakened substantially or in conflict with the internal state of the body. When this happens, synchrony with the immediate environment is lost and problems with sleep become more likely. It has not always been necessary to resort to the extremes of subterranean isolation to explore these issues, as there are useful habitable regions above ground which offer extreme variations in environmental and social conditions. The polar regions have been favoured because of their dramatic patterns of light availability from one season to the next. In the southern hemisphere, for example, the sun never sets during the Antarctic summer, in contrast to the almost complete darkness of the winter months.

Conditions are hostile in these areas and they are unlikely to attract large numbers of people, so they provide a unique opportunity for investigating how the internally driven mechanisms of the body clock cope when faced with an impoverished environment and a totally unfamiliar daily pattern of natural light and dark. In the early 1950s Dr Lewis and Dr Lobban, researchers from the University of Cambridge, England, showed that it was possible to re-adjust the body clock to an artificial day length (shorter or longer days, as in the previous example) in these conditions. To achieve this, volunteers were given a wristwatch set to run either slightly faster or slightly slower than normal[3].

For the experiment, the volunteers were all travelling to the remote region of the Arctic circle known as Spitzbergen for the first time. On separate trips, half the group were presented with individual watches set to run fast, so that they ticked off 24 hours in just 21 hours, while the other half were given watches set to run slow, so that 24 hours in fact lasted for a full 27 hours. In the absence of a familiar sunset or sunrise, both groups were found to organize their daily and nightly activities around the timing of their watches. It seems likely that they were able to do this because their environment lacked clues that would normally conflict with their 'watch-time'. Instead, as there was nothing to suggest otherwise, the time given by the watch was taken on good faith, and the unusual day lengths presented few problems.

'Polar' insomnia

Early experience of isolated research stations suggested that these conditions were problematic and had a direct impact on the sleep of their temporary residents. From the 1970s onwards, a number of experiments were set up to monitor the physical and mental status of volunteers throughout their four to five month stay. Many were found to develop what was to become known as a 'polar insomnia' shortly after their arrival at the base. They would typically report difficulties in getting off to sleep, disruptions during the night and waking up in the morning feeling weary and unrefreshed. Their EEG records confirmed in many cases that the amount of time spent in the deeper stages of sleep and also in dream-related sleep was substantially reduced, to be replaced by lighter and more disturbed sleep.

These findings were interesting for a number of reasons. Firstly, they offered some insight into how much the volunteers relied on the influence of powerful zeitgebers such as natural sunlight in order to maintain a healthy and reliable rhythm of sleep and wake behaviour. Secondly, they also highlighted the importance of a vast range of factors, other than zeitgebers, which can influence whether people sleep soundly or not.

In particular, the stresses of base life was considered to be an important factor in the development of polar insomnia: these included limited social opportunities, basic living conditions and restricted communications with the world beyond the base. Homesickness and mild depression was common in the early days. Interestingly, as conditions on polar scientific stations improved in terms of comforts and amenities towards the 1980s, sleep was also found to show an improvement. These reports suggest that by adhering to a rigid schedule of activity and recreating familiar surroundings and routines, including social as well as work pursuits, it may be possible to counter the more dramatic changes in sleep behaviour resulting from the absence of the predictable daily rising and setting of the sun. Although it helps to have a stark contrast between day and night, this can be achieved to some extent by more artificial means and allows some degree of flexibility for rescheduling just when that 'night' should be.

How important is light?

Some people are more sensitive to changes in light availability than others. Even moderate changes in daylight hours, as with the natural transitions between the seasons, have been associated with changes in sleep patterns and may be an important causative factor in a condition known as Seasonal Affective Disorder (SAD). The symptoms of SAD range from a mild but persistent negative mood (sometimes known as winter blues) to a severe depression which can last for months and lifts only as spring approaches. Sufferers typically eat more, sleep more and are less active during the winter months (when there is less natural daylight) than during the summer. There is some evidence to show that people in the northern hemisphere are more susceptible. In severe cases, it may be possible to treat this condition success-fully using lengthy exposures to artificial bright light, as a substitute for the reduction in available natural light.

Questions for the future

Apart from scientific curiosity, partial or complete 'isolation' studies can help in developing an understanding of our ability to cope with the more extreme demands of modern living. Working the night shift, for example, means that it is necessary to sleep during the day. Because the cues in the environment (daylight, social activity, meal times, noise etc) are all 'out of step' with the will to sleep, this is not always easy to achieve. 'Jet lag' resulting from travel across time zones presents similar problems, including lethargy and insom-nia, sometimes lasting for days, before the body is finally adjusted to the new environment. For those on rotating shift schedules and frequent travellers, lengthy adaptation periods are often difficult to cope with.

Spaceflight

An extreme example of this is faced by astronauts during extended periods in space, when performance and efficiency are all-important, and the problems arising from inadequate sleep need to be kept in careful check. It is now rec-ognized as vital for crew to be able to sleep well during space missions in order to avoid the likely impact of poor sleep on decision-making and response capacity in such a demanding environment.

Although the very early space missions were too short for sleep to be an issue, the first opportunity to try sleep in space came during a Soviet flight in the mid-1960s. Initial observations of actual quality of sleep in space (on the Gemini missions, for example) suggested that astronauts were definitely not sleeping as well as on the ground. But these missions were still relatively short, lasting days rather than months, and difficulty in sleeping was no doubt influenced by extreme psychological stresses.

With the move towards extended space missions and semi-permanent 'sta-tions' such as Skylab, Salyut and Mir, the cumulative effects of sleep problems during missions of 300 days plus became a significant concern for space agencies. The emerging pattern of sleep in space resembled the 'overwinter-ing' problems in the earlier polar studies, with astronauts experiencing less overall sleep, an increase in light, superficial sleep over deep sleep, less dream-ing sleep, and problems with sleep continuity throughout the night.

Returning to earth after long stays on the Mir and Skylab space stations has also been linked with marked difficulties in returning to a normal sleep pattern. Psychological factors following such a stressful event may again be important here.

In addition, spaceflight presents a number of unique sleep problems, many of which stem from the demands imposed by zero gravity inside the spacecraft; the substitution of an unfamiliar pattern of light and darkness; constant noise, vibration and discomfort; and the ongoing psychological stresses of the job:

Zero gravity

• Although 'space motion sickness' is not readily explained, it seems likely that changes in body weight, perception and movement produce conflicting information for a system trained to expect earth's gravity, leading to extended bouts of nausea.
• Some crew members do not mind their arms floating upwards during sleep, while others can only sleep if their arms are secured within a specially designed sleep bag, which is anchored to prevent further movement.
• It has been suggested that during extended missions a rotating working and sleeping area would help to simulate normal gravity, but the technical obstacles to this are prohibitive.

It has been possible to simulate sleeping in zero gravity on earth by sleeping with the head tilted downwards at an angle of 6 degrees. This method has been useful in crew preparation and also for learning more about the effects of zero gravity on the body. In order for it to be effective, however, it is necessary to maintain this position for lengthy periods of time (weeks rather than days).

Light

• Unusual patterns of light fail to regulate the internal body clock. For example, during orbital flights the sun rises and sets about 16 times in every 24-hour period.
• Confusion can be minimized by keeping to 'mission control time' throughout the flight.
• The polar regions have again been useful for training because of their unusual light conditions.
• Attempts are made to adjust the astronauts to the timing of their expected on-board work schedule (whether this is night or whether this is day work) before take-off.

Noise, vibration and comfort

• There is constant noise and vibration of the spacecraft.
• Disturbance arises from crew members on an alternative work schedule.
• Physical activity is limited.
• Conditions are overcrowded.

Psychological stress

• Such stresses are particularly during lengthy missions.
• There is limited social contact and opportunity for recreation.
• There is also limited communication with earth.
• Boredom becomes a factor due to lack of variation.
• Stress is caused by the intensive workload.
• There are problems associated with sleeping and waking in an unfamiliar environment.
• Inevitably, there is anxiety during the critical first few days of a mission.

It has been fairly common for astronauts to use powerful sleeping medications in order to ensure that their limited time for sleep during a mission is used effectively. This is not an ideal solution for a number of reasons:

• Dosage levels for sleeping pills can be unreliable, due to the effects of zero gravity on absorption through the digestive system.
• The residual 'hang-over' effect experienced by many people compromises early-morning efficiency.
• Response to an emergency during the night is jeopardized.

The alternative to medication for tackling the problem of sleep during extended spaceflight is to reproduce, as far as possible, the familiar zeitgebers which convince the body to remain on a 24-hour schedule. The longer the mission, the more difficult this becomes.

A trip to Mars?

There is a popular conviction that Mars represents our best local chance of finding evidence of extra-terrestrial life forms. Fuelled by the first close-up Martian pictures relayed by Mariner 4 in 1965, and the recent Pathfinder surface excursions of the 1990s, the possibility of landing a human being on Mars has gripped the public's imagination. It has been argued that the technology for this will be available within the next 25 years. Although there are no confirmed plans for a mission at present, the opportunity to send a human crew to Mars presents intriguing problems for the sleep scientist.

The major technical obstacles to a trip to Mars involve equipping a spacecraft with sufficient oxygen, fuel, water, food, etc for the return trip. But what are the human problems? A two-year round trip, incorporating time for exploration, has been proposed as a conservative estimate (the 'unmanned' exploration craft Pathfinder took over seven months to get to Mars in 1997). During this time:

• The crew will have to come to terms with an unwieldy communication delay with earth; as they move further out into space, conversations between the crew and mission control will be interrupted by a delay of up to 20 minutes between transmission and reception.
• The physical problems of long-term exposure to zero gravity and the level of psychological stress are unknown, but are likely to be substantial.

• Knowing that contingency plans in the event of an emergency are limited, and with little practical support from earth, the crew are pretty much on their own.

In all, this presents a dramatic reduction of social and environmental zeitgebers, in which the chances of maintaining normal or adequate sleep patterns are slim. It is possible that this factor alone will compromise the effectiveness of the entire mission.

Further down the line, the prospects of adapting to colonial life on Mars are more encouraging, assuming that the problems of radiation, extreme cold and an atmosphere consisting of 95 per cent carbon dioxide can be dealt with. Like the earth, Mars is tilted on its axis and is therefore 'seasonal' in terms of climactic change. On earth, these changes have been useful in synchronizing the body's internal processes with the environment. Given sufficient social zeitgebers, the slightly extended Martian 'day' length, about 37 minutes longer than the earth's, should pose no real problem for the human circadian system.

Today's world

The aim of this chapter has been to give a flavour of the sorts of questions being asked about human sleep patterns and the research strategies that have been developed over the years. For the future, the ability to extend our activities beyond the conventional day/night pattern may well depend on how far we are able to understand, and if necessary control, the complex interaction between the internal and external processes governing sleep.

Until recently, we could predict that for most people the timing of their decision to sleep would be governed by the hours of natural light and dark. In today's world, this is no longer the case.

Chapter 2
A cultural obsession

From time to time, dead people visit my dreams, although my own religious and cultural training tells me not to take this too seriously; this is simply my imagination playing tricks, reconstructing familiar images from the past. It is wishful thinking – I miss them. They are not visiting 'souls', bearing messages from a future life or warnings of imminent danger, but are more likely the result of the complex interactions between psychological and physiological processes which dictate how I feel at any particular moment. Modern scientific advances suggest that in the not too distant future it may be possible to show that the dream 'memory' is nothing more than a reconstruction of a unique pattern of electro-chemical activity across the brain. And yet to be so dismissive of these types of dreams is a relatively new position, and one not shared by everybody.

While scientists have only recently turned their attention to sleep, there are many historic references to suggest that sleep has played an important role in cultural life over the centuries. In *The Golden Bough*[1], a renowned study of magical and religious beliefs published towards the end of the nineteenth century, Sir James Frazer described a remarkable similarity in the interpretation of dreams across primitive cultures from remote areas of the world. One of the more enduring themes to be found was the idea that sleep provides a bridging state between the material, earthly world, and another, perhaps magical or spiritual world. Thus the dream was simply a memory of an encounter with another world, one devoid of all physicality and frequently travelled by the soul after separation from the body at the start of sleep. No doubt it made perfect sense to assume that the soul simply slipped out of the body, perhaps through a facial cavity, and returned shortly before waking. This belief in an existence beyond the physical world is epitomized further by the many religious or mythical stories of apocalyptic or prophetic dreams.

It is only since we have developed a more rational picture of the imagination, in relation to the limitations of the material world, that we now expect to find explanations for what is going on during sleep and dreaming in purely physical terms. Outside forces are no longer a realistic consideration for the modern, scientific view of the origins or functions of dreaming.

On the other hand, at a more popular level there has been a definite reluctance to give up on these 'magical' properties, or to view sleep from a purely rational and scientific perspective. Even nowadays, with an imperative (in most developed societies) to explain all aspects of human behaviour in more earth-bound, physical terms, sleep is nevertheless regarded by many as a unique and mysterious state. There is still enormous support, for example, for the prophetic dream (see Chapter 10) and the out-of-body experience during sleep (see Chapter 11).

If this is the popular, modern view of sleep and dreaming, then there are many interesting parallels to be drawn with beliefs throughout the ages. Ideas that have been around for some time are echoed in modern folklore, reinforced by the ongoing enthusiasm for sleep to be something other than a purely physical experience. A number of recurring themes spring to mind:

• The dream as a pathway to another world.
• Sleep as a release, an escape – perhaps even death.
• Sleep as vulnerable – an 'empty shell'.
• The dream as wish-fulfilment – revealing the true nature of self.
• Sleep as a reflection of character.

Pathway to another world

Although we may be less willing nowadays to credit dreams with a social function, for many early cultures, they played an important role in regulating social behaviours and customs. At the heart of these beliefs was the idea that the soul was released from the body during sleep and was free to wander the earth without normal physical constraints. In some cases, the imagery of the dream was thought to relate to actual events witnessed by the soul during the time it was away from the body. It was quite reasonable, therefore, for the events of a dream to be taken extremely seriously; perhaps as an indication of a neighbouring threat or related danger, in which case counter-strategies would be devised. Similarly, dreams have also been understood as good luck omens. For these reasons, spiritual and community leaders would often look to the dreams of sensitive individuals for guidance. This idea of a privileged few being receptive to dreams relating to the fate of the community led to many elaborate dream 'induction' rituals, perhaps sleeping within the confines of a sacred place or in drug-induced, trance-like states.

Separation of the soul from the physical body was also considered by many to be an extremely vulnerable state. To prevent the soul from losing its way while separated, it was often thought to be attached to the body by some form of umbilical connection, a silver thread or cord being a popular image (this idea is still very popular during the 'modern' out-of-body experience). If, for some reason, the soul was prevented from reuniting with the body, then the individual would be in great peril. Thus there would often be great concern over facilitating this reunion. Sudden awakenings, for example, were thought to be particularly dangerous, leading to insanity or illness, as the soul would not have time to return to the body before full consciousness was established. It was also considered of vital importance for the body of the sleeping person to be in exactly the same posture and location as when the soul departed. This also applied to changes in physical appearance, where the malicious act of daubing make-believe features on the face of a sleeping person could render that person unrecognizable and therefore in grave danger of having their soul cast off forever.

These beliefs formed part of a highly developed system of ideas based on what was known at the time about the material world. They would seem reasonable and were given credence by experience and observation: dreams are realistic, both in sight and sound, and often focus on acts of aggression and violence between known enemies. The general lack of responsiveness of the 'body' during sleep is also consistent with the idea of an 'empty shell' (see page 29), vacated for the duration of sleep.

Release and escape

Sleep has been used in both ancient and modern folklore to provide a release or escape from a less than ideal situation. A recurring theme in both adult and children's literature is the idea of falling asleep for an indefinite period, or at least until more favourable conditions prevail. The protagonists are literally waiting for their 'time' to come. For the Sleeping Beauty, this was the kiss of a handsome prince (Perrault, 1697).

Notice how time stands still for the Sleeping Beauty, preserving her natural and youthful beauty despite the passing of the years. Although we frequently hear the expression 'beauty sleep', the association between sleep and beauty has no obvious scientific history. In Greek mythology Selene, goddess of the moon, was so moved by the beauty of a young shepherd boy, Endymion, that she is said to have drugged him into a state of eternal sleep – although alternative accounts suggest that Endymion initiated his own sleep stasis out of vanity.

In *Rip Van Winkle*, Irvin Washington tells the story of a hen-pecked husband who disappears one day into the Catskill Mountains and is not seen again for over 20 years. On returning to his village, he is mystified to find that he recognizes no one. As far as he is concerned, he had only been away for a single night, after inadvertently falling asleep on the side of the mountain the night before. With gradual realization, it becomes clear to him that 20 years have passed without his knowledge, the only comfort for him being to find out that his wife had died during the intervening years! He rejoices in the release from matrimony and looks forwards to a peaceful life from then on. The story of Rip Van Winkle as a 'sleeper' waiting for better times also has political undercurrents relating to the fight for American Independence.

The Seven Sleepers of Ephesus follows a similar pattern. This story was especially popular in the late Middle Ages, and tells how seven young men, with the help of God, fought back against the oppression of a powerful dictator, Decius, Emperor of Constantinople around 300AD. The story begins with the emperor rejecting the idea of a single, omnipotent God, demanding that his people do the same and join him in the worship of pagan idols. Each citizen must pledge their allegiance to the emperor, and publicly denounce their faith in God, or accept the penalty of death.

Seven young men come forward and express their difficulties with the Emperor's request. Although he feels bound to carry out his threat, the Emperor is reluctant to do so because the men are all of noble birth, and he feels a certain fondness for them. They are allowed time to reconsider their position. During this time, the men are extremely worried and hide in a mountain cave on the outskirts of the city.

As the time for them to repent approaches, the emperor sends out a search party who, on discovering their whereabouts, block the entrance of the cave with rocks, sentencing the seven young men to almost certain death. One of the workers, not happy with what is taking place, decides to leave details of the emperor's actions carved on a stone tablet, which he then hides inside the entrance to the cave. By this time, all the men inside have fallen into a deep sleep.

One hundred years later, the cave is re-opened by a local farmer. The seven young men wake up and one of them is elected to put on a disguise and go into the city to buy food. The traders, however, do not recognize the currency of his coins and become suspicious of the stranger, believing him to have found a valuable treasure. The alarm is raised and the young man is brought before the city's bishop, where he describes how he and his friends were forced to hide from Decius in the caves. The bishop is not unsympathetic to the young man's distress and his insistence that his parents (whom the bishop knows to be long dead) live within the city limits. The bishop and a party of townspeople agree to accompany him back to the cave to his waiting friends. At the entrance to the cave, the tablet of stone left by the workman is found. Breaking the seal, the details of the persecution by Decius and the blocking of the entrance to the cave are read out to the waiting crowd. It becomes clear that over 100 years have since passed and Decius had died many years before. The bishop declares a miracle and the faith of the seven young men is celebrated throughout the city.

As with Rip Van Winkle, the seven 'sleepers' of Ephesus felt as if they had been asleep for just one night, and on waking they are amazed to find everything they once knew is now gone. They are actually displaced in time through sleep to a better, more peaceful period.

We have modern equivalents to these stories, mainly through films, in which the protagonist finds an escape through sleep. In *Forever Young*, starring Mel Gibson and popular in the mid-1980s, the main character 'sleeps' in suspended animation after being traumatized by the events of his waking life. When he is finally reawakened decades later, his optimism for life gradually returns. In *Sleeper*, the Woody Allen character makes a similar shift in time after a lengthy sleep. Throughout these stories the world goes on in the background, while the 'sleeper' waits for something better to come along.

An 'empty shell'

Sleep has also been seen as a period of vulnerability, with the idea in many ancient cultures that the body is temporarily abandoned by the spirit or soul of a person during sleep (signified by the lack of responsiveness) and left in a vulnerable or dangerous state. Many elaborate behaviours were therefore devised to ward off danger during sleep.

It is not simply a question of physical powerlessness during sleep and dulled response to danger, but an altogether more sinister vulnerability through which we are exposed to events even scarier than earthly dangers. For the soul travellers, it was the fear of not being able to return to the body at the end of the sleep, perhaps because the body had been moved or disguised, or because the soul was waylaid during the night.

This vulnerability during sleep is recognized in many traditional and modern popular stories. Bram Stoker's famous novel *Dracula* (1897) was based largely on traditional stories of blood-sucking, evil creatures, known as vampires, who preyed on humans during sleep by literally sucking out their life-blood. Samson lost his strength after Delilah cut his hair while he was asleep. In *Jack and the Beanstalk*, the giant's golden hen is literally stolen from under his nose while he sleeps. Ironically, even the vampire is powerless during sleep, an event he is unable to forestall with the rising of the sun.

In cinema, the idea of being defenceless during sleep, particularly to a malevolent force, is a hugely successful horror theme. Sleep is also a period of sinister metamorphosis, as with the transformation of Bram Stoker's Lucy from virgin to vampire. In *The Midwich Cuckoos* (filmed as *Village of the Damned*) the residents of an entire village are 'taken over' by aggressive alien visitors as they sleep. In the *The Bodysnatchers*, a similar fate awaited San Francisco residents, whose only chance of survival was to stay awake indefinitely.

Sleep also provides the ultimate escape and is often shown to be closely related to death in terms of physical appearance and temporal proximity. According to Roman mythology, Death and Somnus (the god of sleep) are twin brothers, both sons of Night. In the story of Romeo and Juliet, William Shakespeare showed how easy it would be to mistake these two. Despite agreeing on a fake suicide, Romeo was so convinced by Juliet's induced deep slumber that he believed she was dead, and took his own life.

The true nature of self

Dreams have always provided an important source of validation for social taboos and superstitions, the significance of which has not declined despite the move towards more complex, organized societies. For example, the dream played an important role in Greek, Nordic and Roman mythologies. For the Greeks, the dream provided a channel for communication between gods and mortals. Advice, commands and cures for serious illness or infertility were all typical dream topics. The Egyptians were also fastidious in recording and monitoring dream content. The dream is central to many New and Old Testament stories of apocalyptic prophecies or divine intervention.

This can present something of a dilemma for today's schoolchildren, who are expected to accept the reality of premonitions and visitations during dreams in the contexts of these stories, but are then told on a more day-to-day level that these events do not happen in 'modern' dreams. Until fairly recently, beliefs about the potential of dreaming were all premised on the assumption of forces beyond the physical acting on the mind of the 'dreamer' during sleep, and visions or premonitions were invariably concerned with physical events – such as a flood, illness or other risk. Today's preoccupation is with the psychological significance of the dream.

Although it is difficult to pinpoint the shift towards a more scientific understanding of the processes taking place during sleep, there were clear signs of this happening in the writing of European and American medical professions towards the end of the nineteenth century. At this time, few doubted that sleep was an essential process for the human body, although how this might be achieved generated fierce debate. Suggestions that sleep had some function at the level of the brain cell (the neuron), perhaps to allow the cleansing of fatigue-related substances that built up in the cell during wakefulness, were on the increase. There was also growing support for the idea that sleep effected some sort of emotional recovery or rest.

A turning point in the history of popular ideas about sleep and dreaming was reached around the turn of the century with the work of Sigmund Freud. Having first trained as a medical doctor, throughout his later life Freud developed – and became famous for – a method of treating psychological disturbances based on a technique known as psychoanalysis. He argued that the dream was of immense importance in understanding the root of individual, emotional and psychological disturbance.

At the heart of this technique was the assumption that the mind operates on different levels of awareness, and that clues to the ideas and thoughts which are too disturbing for us to deal with at the conscious level could be found within the content of a dream. The purpose of psychoanalysis was to employ techniques to unearth the roots of emotional turmoil, and the extraction of the true meaning from the elaborate and ambiguous symbolism of the dream experience was considered to be particularly useful in this regard.

For Freud, many of the preoccupations and emotional concerns of adult life could be traced to earlier, childhood experiences. Although criticized for his emphasis on sexual motivations, Freud maintained that many of the fears, anxieties and obsessions of his patients could be traced back to conflicts between basic, 'primitive' drives and the recognition and desire to conform to social mores. However, although internalized at the subconscious level, these conflicts continue to have a powerful influence on thought processes and behaviour in everyday life. The concept of repression, through which these conflicts are prevented from invading our conscious thoughts, is crucial to this theory. While the conscious mind is thought to turn away from unpleasant or unpalatable thoughts or recollections, as a form of self-protection, such issues are addressed indirectly through the latent (or hidden) content of the dream. So conflicts which we may not be willing to recognize and explore in our waking experience are 'censored' from consciousness, but may be present themselves (following transformation) in our dreams. Thus the dream acts as a kind of 'safety valve' for feelings of guilt, fear, hostility, anger and aggression stemming from unresolved emotional conflict.

This was to be an important development in the medical and popular conception of dreams; while the surreal nature of the dream had previously lent support to the idea of its being 'other-worldly' and externally generated, Freud argued that the dream was nothing more than the constructions of the imagination. He was dismissive of primitive accounts of the dream, described by him as the 'mythological hypothesis' on dreaming, which failed to realize the power of the human mind in generating dream phenomena without recourse to outside forces (whether divine or magical). This recognition – that all dreaming occurred inside the head – was a critical turning point, signalling as it did the adoption of the dream by the scientific, medical world and thus rendering it open to systematic inspection.

Despite much initial criticism from within the medical profession, the psychoanalytic approach gathered momentum in the aftermath of World War I, having proved an exciting and innovative approach to the problem of how to treat 'shell-shocked' soldiers returning from the front lines of battle.

By the mid-1940s the idea that the dream could be used to unlock the secrets of the inner-working mind was no longer confined to the scientific or medical fields, but was beginning to filter out to a more popular level. The tantalizing suggestion of self-knowledge and a developing fascination for the mysteries of the mind fuelled public interest in this area – an interest which was soon to be recognized within the world of popular entertainment.

In his classic movie thriller *Spellbound*, starring Gregory Peck and Ingrid Bergman, Alfred Hitchcock introduced the more glamorous and intriguing aspects of these ideas to a wider audience. *Spellbound* told the story of a man who turns up at a psychiatric institute with no memory of his past life, only to be mistaken for a psychiatrist who was due to arrive at around the same time. However, his lack of expertise soon alerts the suspicions of the resident psychiatrist. She is not unsympathetic, though, and agrees to help him when he confesses that he has absolutely no idea who he is or where he has come from, only an overwhelming sense of foreboding.

The man's amnesia is quickly identified as trauma-related and the bona fide psychiatrist sets out to get to the bottom of things through dream analysis. This is followed by a now famous dream sequence, as the amnesic man describes the imagery and content of his recent disturbing dream. The psychiatrist explains that the bizarre imagery of the dream represents codified references to thoughts or events that are buried deep within his subconscious. Through a process of systematic interpretation, she is able to reveal the true meaning of the dream and so help the man face the trauma which led to his amnesia. In this way, he is able to address the truth of recent events, and his memory returns instantly (and miraculously).

Of course, the time constraints of the film glossed over the lengthy psychoanalytic process, which under normal circumstances would be extremely unlikely to prompt an instant 'cure' on the basis of a single dream. *Spellbound* was nevertheless important, because for perhaps the first time a large section of the public was introduced to the idea that dreams are important for emotional stability, and also that the mind is capable of holding back, ie having secrets.

With *Spellbound*, Hitchcock recognized the value of the dream in firing the imagination and made contemporary scientific ideas accessible to the viewing public. The dream has since become an extremely popular device for the film-maker and dramatist for a number of reasons, not least being the freedom from the restraints of a sequential time series offered by the dream 'cliché', in which the plot shifts between real and imagined events. It is now a familiar theme in cinema, and reinforces a more general perception that through the dream, experts can literally help you to 'know your own mind'. This has also coincided with widespread acceptance of the psychoanalytic approach to mental health, and the development of a conventional wisdom that the dream offers to share important secrets of the psyche. To understand the dream is to know the self.

This idea that we can know ourselves or be known through dreams is a familiar one in modern literature. In Victorian London, Charles Dickens used dreams to reacquaint Scrooge with his own conscience. In *Finnegan's Wake*, James Joyce explored the motivations of his central character through a series of dreams. In the 1950s, Dylan Thomas used the idea of dreams to great effect in *Under Milk Wood*, exposing, through the course of a single night, the intimate secrets and desires of the residents of a sleepy Welsh fishing village.

Wish-fulfilment

Freud popularized the idea of the dream as a disguised wish, in which we allude to objects of desire which may otherwise be beyond our grasp, or morally or socially unacceptable. He described a series of developmental stages, reflecting a 'natural' sequence of social and moral development in which we are gradually made aware of the forbidden nature of certain basic pleasures. It is argued that because we each go through a similar process, this produces similarities in dreams at the various stages. Central to this idea is the preoccupation with family relationships, representing as they do the earliest exposure to social mores and a repression of egotistical drives.

So at the heart of the dream lies the truth of who and what we are, and what it is that we desire. It is clear that these ideas have had an enormous impact on the popular understanding of a dream, whether through transparent desire or as a route to the subconscious. In language, the dream is now synonymous with legitimate desire and provides powerful rhetoric: as with Dr Martin Luther King's famous civil rights speech, in which he declared, 'I have a dream...'. It is difficult to imagine 'I have a plan...' or 'I have an idea...' carrying the same weight. Similarly, the idea of the American Dream invokes an individual claim to freedom to follow one's dreams based on opportunity. As such, dreaming is now considered to be not simply a normal but also an essential feature of both sleep and wake.

Reflection of character

If dreaming represents the glamorous 'mental' side of sleep, there has always been a suspicion that we can do without the physical process, given the right attitude. At times we have toyed with pushing the limits of endurance without sleep to extremes. During the Depression, for example, dance marathons were popular in the USA. These events, with prizes often in excess of $1,000 for the last couple dancing, offered solutions to unemployment and poverty. It has been claimed that the record for this was 5,148 hours (although dancers were generally allowed 15 minutes' break each hour), before a number of deaths led to the authorities discouraging further competitions.

The idea that sleep can say something about the type of person you are dates back to at least the Middle Ages. The following proverbs and sayings were compiled in the sixteenth to seventeenth centuries[2-4], although a few are still around in modern equivalents. Many of these reflect distaste for over-indulgence in sleep, while demonstrating amazing insight into the physiological sleep process. For example, the influence of internal functions, particularly digestion, on dreaming was already suspected:

When a man sleeps his head is in his stomach.

So was the existence of biological rhythms or patterns in sleep:

In the morning... there happen more pleasant and certeine [certain] dreams.

This particular proverb (dating back to before 1584) shows an awareness of differences between sleep states throughout the night that have only been confirmed (scientifically) during the last 60–70 years. The fact that we tend to dream more during the later part of the night is now well known and easy to demonstrate with modern techniques. In addition, the awareness of more 'pleasant' dreams towards the morning suggests an early recognition of the nightmares of deep sleep (common in the first one or two hours of the night).

The dream was also recognized as an unrealized wish:

We see sleeping that which we wish for waking.
What man desires in the day, he dreames in the night.

There are also many examples in which sleep patterns are considered to reflect on the character of the individual. These tend to emphasize the value of going without sleep and a growing intolerance for excessive sleep:

One slumber invites another.
The more a man sleeps, the more he may.
The sleepy fox has seldom feathered breakfast.

On the other hand, it has long been realized that:

The early bird catches the worm.

And that peace of mind is essential for sound sleep:

A quiet conscience sleeps in thunder.

Early proverbs also show an acute awareness of natural body rhythms:

One hour's sleep before midnight is worth two after.

In this respect, 'larks' were already favoured over 'owls' (see also Chapter 6):

To watch in the moon and sleep in the sun is neither profit nor honour.
He who sleeps all the morning may go a-begging all the day after.

The nature of dreams

Finally, at its most bland, the dream has been described as a random series of neuronal firings. Not everybody is convinced. Whereas a cynic might argue that a persistence with pre-scientific beliefs about sleep reflects more general anxieties about the meaning of life, we do not have to look too far to see that for many people, the richness of the dream experience demands an explanation beyond that provided by the mechanics of the brain.

Chapter 3

The modern sleep laboratory

In today's modern sleep laboratory, although there are still many unresolved fundamental questions concerning sleep, there has been a shift in focus towards understanding and managing more contemporary 'sleep' problems. The purpose of this chapter is to give an overview of some of these problems, and the techniques and methods currently being used to further research in this area. Some sleep-related concepts are also introduced to facilitate understanding of information in later chapters.

Certainly, much of the early research into sleep makes for fascinating reading, and gives some idea of the enthusiasm and ingenuity with which researchers approached their subject. Armed with the tools of the relatively new discipline of experimental psychology, sleep was to be re-conceptualized in terms of its physiological functions and its relationship with the waking state. For the early sleep researchers, this often involved subjecting themselves and others to extreme levels of physical and psychological deprivation in their attempts to discover the true reasons for sleep. Their efforts, during the first half of this century, set the scene for future research by identifying what were to become the key issues in this area.

Nowadays, scientists tend to adopt a more pragmatic approach to the reasons for sleep, by asking what sleep research can tell us about how people operate in the 'real world' rather than under laboratory conditions. For this reason, the experimental extremes of sleep loss are unlikely to be repeated. So, what *are* the concerns of the modern sleep laboratory? Although the fundamental questions about sleep are still important and continue to intrigue scientists, the current agenda has been dominated somewhat by more immediate lifestyle problems. However, the two approaches are not mutually exclusive.

Fundamental issues

The questions detailed below are central to our observations concerning sleep and have widespread relevance for a more general understanding of what happens during sleep. They are, quite simply, the $64,000 questions in sleep research.

What happens (to the brain) when we sleep?

Researchers have taken a range of approaches to this question:

• *Describing the chemistry of the brain.* Is there a sleep 'substance' in the brain which builds up to trigger the need for sleep? Can this be found in nature, plants, food? Can it be synthesized in drugs? To date, nothing has been found in humans that might fit the bill.

• *Describing the progressive changes in sleep across the night.* It was clear even without sophisticated techniques that there are qualitative differences in the way that we sleep through the night. Sleep tends to be deeper earlier in the night, and shallower and more prone to disturbance towards the second half of the night. Progress in describing these changes was accelerated by the development of techniques to monitor the brain's activity during sleep (see below).

• *Understanding a tolerance for adjustments in sleep pattern.* How little sleep can a person manage with?

• *Looking at what being asleep means.* Is it a question of total sensory shut-down? This seems unlikely, as there is good evidence that at some points during the night we are processing information from around us and are able to respond, for example, to significant and familiar noises. In fact, the brain is surprisingly active during the dreaming phases of sleep.

• *Exploring the purpose of dreaming.* In the 1960s, researchers were able to relate dream recall and content to specific physiological changes in the brain and the movements of the eyes. Since this time, scientists have attempted to reconcile changes in the chemistry of the brain with the emotional experience of dreaming.

As you can see, although there have been many advances over the years in describing the mechanisms of sleep – ie how we do it – there is still no simple answer to the question of *why* we sleep. The most popular ideas at the moment include:

• The body needs to sleep in order to do something which it cannot do during wake – the obvious candidates for this 'something' include growth or tissue repair, and yet the evidence for this is equivocal.

• Sleep keeps us out of harm's way. We are not physically geared for operating at night, unlike the more successful nocturnal creatures, who cope well in conditions of low visibility and time their own activity to coincide with the availability of natural prey.

• During sleep, the brain performs a 'housekeeping' routine – clearing out old memories, reorganizing new ones, restoring mental alertness, etc.

• Sleep performs a psychological function (during dreaming), perhaps by allowing subconscious conflicts to be addressed.

The primary aims of most current sleep-deprivation experiments are centred around shedding light on the latter two theories (which are not mutually exclusive).

How do we know when to sleep?

This includes such questions as:
• What is the nature of the 'biological clock'?
• How does the daily pattern of sleepiness fit in with other biological rhythms, such as daily fluctuations in temperature?
• What are the effects on mood and cognition?
• How do external factors such as daylight, social activity and knowledge of time affect sleep?
• How powerful is the internal biological rhythm for sleep?
• How do we react to a change in environment, such as a shift in time zones?

Current issues

The last 20–30 years or so have seen a massive increase in the number of people working unusual, long or unpredictable hours, as well as increased automation and urbanization, and all-night traffic noise. These factors have also introduced the problem of how to stay awake outside a normal routine or, in some cases, how to sleep when the body is telling you otherwise.

Scientists working in this area have been keen to tackle these questions head-on, as many of them coincide with a growing concern that a substantial proportion of the world's population is either not getting enough sleep, or is trying to sleep at the wrong time.

Sleep in a modern society

Questions being asked and problems addressed include:
• Are contemporary lifestyles and the sleep patterns of complex, industrial societies incongruous with a natural drive to sleep? Have we lost touch with the needs of the body?
• How can we know if somebody is sleepy? What are the dangers, and who is at risk? Regulations concerning work hours and shift types are constantly under review by legislative bodies. Lately, concerns about the need for sleep and the importance of 'body clock' factors have been gradually introduced into this debate. The urgency for this is reinforced by recent evidence to suggest that a large proportion of road and industrial accidents occur during the vulnerable periods of the daily sleepiness cycle, ie at night and, to a lesser extent, in mid-afternoon.
• Is sleepiness dangerous? How long should a person be allowed to continue working in an emergency situation without sleep? The conventional wisdom seems to be that the decision-makers of the world can pull themselves together under pressure and deal with anything that is thrown at them, whereas all the evidence suggests that this is simply not the case. After staying up all night, rather than being on top form you are more likely to be inflexible, arrogant, unimaginative and inarticulate.

• How can we ensure peaceful, restful sleep? What are the problems of living in built-up areas? Why can some people tolerate aircraft flying overhead, traffic and train noise during sleep, while others cannot?

• Sleep medicine – there have been enormous advances in the identification and treatment of disorders associated with sleep, such as sleep apnoea, narcolepsy, and insomnia.

• Shiftwork – what happens when we make repeated adjustments to sleep patterns?

• Jet lag – how can we overcome a sudden transition between time zones, when the body and the outside world disagree over when it is time for you to sleep? This has particular relevance for the military and business worlds, where the need is to limit the time taken to re-synchronize over time zones so that personnel can perform at peak levels immediately or soon after arrival.

Studying sleep: methods and techniques

While earlier investigations into sleep had to rely to a great extent on the observations of the experimenter or the introspection of the volunteers, the modern sleep laboratory is equipped with an impressive and sophisticated range of tools for measuring all aspects of sleep. Some of these are appropriate for field work (which can involve a large number of volunteers), while others are the preferred method for use in the laboratory. The decision to make use of a particular technique will depend almost entirely on the number of people involved, how much you need to know about their sleep, the number of nights you wish to monitor their sleep, and the extent to which you think they are able to tolerate the use of invasive equipment (a factor particularly relevant in the case of the very young, the very old and ill volunteers).

Methods for monitoring sleep can be categorized broadly into objective or subjective measures. Objective measures produce quantifiable information which can tell us about the physiology of the sleep process, while subjective measures can give us an insight into the sleep process as it is experienced. Objective measures tend to be more expensive than subjective measures, because of the cost of the equipment involved and the demands made on human resources. On the other hand, subjective measures might involve nothing more than filling in a form regularly, and this approach can often yield valuable information at relatively low cost.

The electroencephalogram (EEG)

Many significant advances in sleep research have relied on the use of the electroencephalogram (EEG) for monitoring the activity of the brain during sleep. This is a painless procedure, which involves fixing small, coated electrodes at specific points across the scalp and measuring changes in electrical potential relayed from the surface of the brain. These can then be plotted out on a very small time frame to trace second-by-second changes in the level of activity and produce a familiar 'brain wave' pattern on a paper record.

The technique was developed originally in the 1920s by Hans Berger in Germany and has since been an invaluable clinical tool for detecting abnormalities in brain function. Around the 1940s, however, it was used during a normal night's sleep. A number of observations which had been made earlier without the benefit of this technique were to be confirmed. Most important of these concerned changes in sleep 'depth' through the night. Just from observations, it was clear that there are differences in breathing, movement and responsiveness from the beginning to the end of the night's sleep. Specifically, the ease with which a person can be woken from sleep and restored to full alertness improves as the night goes on. Added to this, it was clear that following a lengthy period of sleep loss, a person will rapidly descend into deep, unresponsive sleep. This all suggested that sleep, rather than being a uniform state, could be broken down into a number of specific stages.

With the benefit of the EEG it was possible to show that brain activity during a normal night's sleep follows a distinct and universal pattern from one person to the other. These observations formed the foundation of what was to become a widely accepted system of describing sleep.

The EEG is now one of the most popular and revealing techniques for monitoring sleep and is widely relied upon in modern sleep research, where it has applications for both clinical and basic research. Its appeal lies with being able to provide an insight into the brain's activity during sleep. Considerable effort has been targeted into relating the emerging patterns with a subjective experience of what it is like to be asleep, and what, if anything, we are capable of during this period.

Sleep stages

A number of distinct types or 'stages' of sleep can be identified in the EEG. Interestingly, the progression between stages across the night is quite uniform. This led to a 'system' of recording sleep based on the sleep stage indicated by the EEG at any particular point in the night. Thus it was possible to build up a clear picture of 'normal' sleep, a profile which was to be particularly useful in assessing sleep disorders and the effects of any experimental manipulation, such as lengthening, shortening or rescheduling sleep.

It is possible to classify the sleep EEG into one of five basic sleep stages:
• *Stage 1* This is fairly light sleep, usually occurring at the transition points between wake and sleep states. In contrast with the erratic waking EEG, during the descent into sleep the first stages are indicated by a gradual slowing of the EEG. Occasionally during this stage the eyeballs roll gently under closed

lids. Although this is classified as sleep, there would be little difficulty in waking a person from this stage, and, when it occurs at the start of the night, it is possible that they will have no recollection of being asleep unless they were in Stage 1 for longer than a minute or so. Under normal conditions, we spend only a matter of minutes each night in Stage 1.

• *Stage 2* This represents a more established state of sleep – the EEG shows a distinct, non-ambiguous pattern of waves. Muscle tension is beginning to dissolve and the eyes are now still. To the observer, individuals in Stage 2 would probably appear sound asleep. They are less responsive to noise than during Stage 1, and may easily sleep thorough the occasional door banging. Stage 2 occupies about half the night's sleep for a normal night.

• *Stage 3* This is quite sound sleep. The EEG shows a distinct pattern of rolling, slow waves far removed from the chaos of the waking EEG. Muscle tone is still low and the eyes are still.

• *Stage 4* This is considered to be the deepest, least responsive state of sleep. Stages 3 and 4 are often considered together and can be described as Slow Wave Sleep or Delta sleep. We would normally expect to spend less than a quarter of a night in either stage 3 or stage 4 sleep.

• *Stage 5 Rapid Eye Movement (REM)* (Pronounced to rhyme with 'them') Because of its association with dreaming, this is probably considered by many to be the most exciting stage of sleep. The link was made in the 1950s, when it was observed that from time to time during sleep the eyes would become activated under closed lids, moving about in a frenetic, random pattern within the socket. When woken during this phase, volunteers would be far more likely to report being in the middle of a dream than at other stages when the eyes were still. Although the popular understanding of REM sleep is that it is synonymous with the process of dreaming, it appears that dreaming is not limited to this stage but can also taken place at other times during sleep. REM sleep occupies about a quarter of a night for the average, normal night.

One theory of REM sleep emphasizes its role in memory consolidation. Experientially, REM dreaming is perhaps considered by many people to be the most significant aspect of sleep.

Because REM sleep is also signalled by distinct changes in muscle tone and eye movements, in addition to the scalp electrodes it is usual to place electrodes over muscle groups, such as the chin area and around the eyes, to help identify when an individual is in this stage of sleep.

In addition to these five sleep stages, the EEG also records brief periods of wake or semi-arousal from time to time throughout the night.

NREM or REM sleep

A broad distinction is made between what is known as REM sleep, and non-REM or NREM sleep (Stages 1–4 inclusive). It became clear early on that the two states represented very different types of sleep. During REM sleep the mind and brain are extremely active, with most of our narrative-type dreams occurring during these periods. In contrast to all this activity, the body is effectively paralysed to prevent the physical acting-out of the dream content. This restraint on activity is only temporary. In contrast, there are far fewer dreams reported following NREM sleep and no body paralysis. (Interestingly, dreams that do occur during NREM sleep tend to be of a different nature, often more terrifying or emotional – see Chapters 11 and 14).

It is a fairly predictable feature of nightly sleep patterns that in healthy adults NREM sleep is concentrated during the early period of the night, with most REM sleep occurring during the second half of the night.

Sleep 'cycles'

Throughout a single night we make frequent shifts between states. This follows a fairly predictable pattern of 'cycles', covering a period of NREM and REM sleep. Each of these cycles lasts for approximately 90 minutes, and is repeated four to five times each night. However, the cycle itself changes in terms of the proportion of NREM to REM sleep as the night progresses. Whereas Stages 3 and 4 sleep dominate the first two sleep cycles, after this point (about three to four hours into sleep) the likelihood of these sleep stages appearing throughout the rest of the night is drastically reduced. In contrast, REM sleep comes into its own towards the end of the night (cycles three to five).

What else happens during sleep?

• Barring unusual scheduling, the *onset of sleep* coincides with a slight drop in body temperature. Pulse rate and blood pressure are also reduced.

• At the *start of REM sleep* there are signs of irregular breathing, and fluctuations in pulse and blood pressure

• We experience *frequent awakenings during the night*, waking up far more often than we actually remember. One of the reasons for this is that we normally have to be awake for at least two minutes before we remember it the next morning.

• The moments *just before waking up* coincide with an increase in body temperature and levels of cortisol. We also become more restless during this period of sleep, moving around more and experiencing brief semi-arousals.

Other techniques for monitoring sleep

In addition to the EEG, there have also been developments in brain imaging techniques which allow a three-dimensional picture of the brain in the sleeping state. However, it is not always feasible or possible to record physiological evidence of sleep and at times the researcher must rely on alternative methods for the collection of data.

Movement sensors

There are a number of devices available which work on the principle that if a person is inactive for a lengthy period of time (and this coincides with corroborative evidence such as hour-by-hour diaries) they are likely to be asleep. In practical terms, it is more likely that a large group of people will be persuaded to wear small movement sensors in order to get some idea of normal activity patterns, rather than have a full set of EEG monitoring equipment on their heads for 24 hours at a time. Although the information from a movement sensor is basic relative to that which can be gained from an EEG recording, it may be the most pragmatic approach under the circumstances. This method works best if it is possible to average recordings across a number of days and so produce a 'typical' day/night profile.

Video telemetry

Another technique which has been found to be effective in monitoring sleep behaviour is that of video telemetry. This allows a visual recording of all movement and behaviours during sleep. It can be particularly useful in assessing the potential for self-harm during sleep-walking episodes, for example. The camera would presumably be as unobtrusive as possible and could be set up in almost any bedroom, in the hospital or in the patient/volunteer's home. This technique is likely to be used in combination with a full EEG recording, so that the activity on the video recording can be synchronized with the exact state of the brain in order to ascertain, for example, whether the person is asleep or awake, in REM or NREM sleep. For these reasons, telemetry is particularly suited to the diagnosis of sleep disorders.

Subjective accounts – sleep diaries

Often, due to time or financial constraints, it is not possible to adopt one of the more 'high-tech' approaches to monitoring sleep. In these circumstances, the more basic subjective measure of asking people to submit their own accounts of their sleeping behaviour can be successful. Volunteers are typically asked to keep a 'diary' of their nightly sleep (see pages 64–6). These are completed first thing in the morning on waking and are organized around basic questions such as:
• What time did you turn off the light?
• Roughly how long did it take you to go to sleep?
• How many times did you wake up during the night?
• What time did you wake up this morning?

Sleep diaries have the advantage over other methods that they can be kept for weeks or even years to give a long-term view, and can be distributed to very large groups of volunteers. The problems arise with the ability to make subjective judgements about sleep. It is not uncommon to find substantial differences in how long somebody thinks it took them to fall asleep and how long they think they slept for, compared with the evidence or 'objective' records provided by the EEG.

The personal account has nevertheless been invaluable in gathering information about population trends. For example, in the late 1960s the American Cancer Society conducted a survey with over one million participants. This was mainly concerned with lifestyles and health and included questions about sleep behaviours, and the outcome was extremely valuable in terms of confirming the seven-and-a-half to eight-hour sleep as the American social norm of the time. It is only with the subjective account that a survey of this scale could be contemplated.

Age-related sleep patterns

Sleep patterns vary widely across the population. Much of this variation can be explained in terms of individuality in sleep requirements. This is influenced to a great extent by time of life. We can probably expect to be poor sleepers at least twice in our lifetime: when we are very young and when we are very old. If we are lucky, between infancy and old age sleep will be fairly trouble free. The development of sleep patterns across the lifespan allows for certain generalizations:

• In the first few days following birth, many babies spend up to two-thirds of the 24-hour period asleep, waking only to feed approximately every two to four hours (but not all! See Chapter 7). At this stage, there is no distinction between night or day for the baby.

• By three to six months the average baby still spends around 12 hours in every 24 sleeping, but may have started to show a preference for being awake during the day and asleep for most of the night. Although sleep is still common during the day, this is more likely during the afternoon period than in the morning. This 'bi-modal' pattern of sleepiness (concentrated around the night and then again in the afternoon) continues throughout a lifetime, although many cultures dissuade older children and adults from succumbing to the typical early-afternoon urge for sleep.

• As a child grows, the amount of time spent in sleep gradually decreases. Many western primary schools expect five-year-old children to have outgrown an afternoon nap on admission, although some pre-school systems may still cater for it.

• The structure of sleep is also markedly different between adults and children. The child's sleep 'cycle' tends to be shorter between the ages of five and ten years – around 60–70 minutes – with the typical adult 90-minute cycle only emerging through the later teen years.

• Older adults often complain of sleeping less, difficulty in falling asleep and maintaining sleep throughout the night, and early-morning awakening. From 60 years onwards people begin to rely more on sleeping pills on a long-term basis. This is a disturbing trend, particularly bearing in mind recent improvements in life expectancy beyond this age. The evidence provides a mixed explanation for the sleep problems of old age. Factors that may have an effect on the ability to sleep soundly at night for this age group are both physical and social in nature. By addressing these areas, it may be possible to achieve satisfactory levels of sleep.

Concepts and terms

At this point it will be helpful to outline some of the concepts used by sleep clinicians and researchers, many of which are used to establish diagnostic criteria or have been important in understanding some of the more pressing problems in society in relation to sleep.

General terms

Circadian rhythms

Many of the body's natural functions are organized around a daily pattern, and are described as following a 'circadian rhythm' (circadian meaning 'around a day'). These include the drive to sleep and to be active, fluctuations in body temperature, digestion and the production of a range of body chemicals which impact on behaviour levels, including adrenalin and cortisol. Taken together, this waxing and waning of physical processes helps to prepare us for action during the day, and restful sleep during the night. In popular terms, we talk about having a 'body clock' and are usually aware of its influence only when we try to fight against it, ie when we are very sleepy. The area of the brain which is influential in maintaining these rhythms is known as the suprachiasmatic nucleus.

Practically all organisms follow a rhythmic behaviour pattern, which persists even when in an alien environment: the earliest experiments in this area date back to the eighteenth century and describe how plants would still raise and lower their leaves each day even when they were placed in darkness.

For humans living in complex, organized social groups the circadian 'day' is fine-tuned to fit in with the external 24-hour day as determined by the powerful influence of natural light and dark, and other 'time-givers' or zeitgebers. Without these clues, the internal body clock has a natural rhythm that is slightly longer – around 24½ hours per day. This would mean an extra half hour of activity at the end of each day and would gradually put us out of synchrony with the natural environment, which favours activity – for humans at least – during the daytime. External factors are therefore important in training the body clock to follow a more convenient time period.

Circadian types: owls and larks

Not everybody follows the same rhythm – most people are aware of certain times of the day and night when they are feeling at their best. At the two extremes, night 'owls' are at a disadvantage first thing in the morning but are able to continue late into the day without flagging, while 'larks' are primed for morning activity but cannot cope so well with late nights.

Free-running experiments

These refer to artificial environments in which time clues are removed and the body is allowed to follow its natural rhythm. Variations on this theme include experiments where an alternative day length is imposed by following a strict time schedule of light, dark, sleeping, waking, eating and behaviour periods.

Hypnotics or sleeping pills

Certain situations require more direct intervention to ensure sleep. Hypnotics or sleeping pills are widely available on prescription (in addition to a range of 'natural' substances claiming to have sedative properties). There are concerns about the difficulty of shaking off drowsiness the next morning and of long-term usage, although many of the modern varieties claim to have addressed these problems. Sleeping difficulties can also benefit from other, non-drug approaches which focus on identifying underlying problems, arising from domestic or emotional circumstances, for example.

Sleep deprivation

Loss of sleep can occur in many forms and for a wide variety of reasons. The very idea of sleep deprivation makes the assumption that we need at least a certain level of sleep, although determining exactly how much this might be is never easy. For example, we can be 'deprived' of sleep simply by deciding to sleep less than we have come to expect through habit, but whether or not this will leave us *physically* deprived of sleep (ie sleeping less than we really need) is open to debate. Conversely, it is suggested that many people are sleep deprived without being aware of it, and despite a fairly regular pattern of nightly sleep. What we have come to see as 'normal' – feeling wretched in the morning and taking regular caffeine 'hits' to get through the day – is seen as further evidence for this. In the laboratory, sleep loss is 'measured' as the difference between an experimental sleep period and an habitual one, ie the number of hours a volunteer would normally sleep.

Sleep loss usually takes the form of acute total sleep deprivation (in which case it is often more accurate to talk of hours of wakefulness) or partial chronic sleep deprivation. Total sleep deprivation is nowadays invariably limited to a matter of nights rather than weeks, and would include, for example, the fairly commonplace experience of staying up all night. At this level, many people find they are able to cope with the experience by staying busy, and will be even more motivated to ignore the discomfort of sleepiness if they have a good reason for staying awake. On the other hand, by the second night, the problems of staying awake are beyond many people's endurance. For these reasons, one night without sleep is a particularly interesting period of sleep loss to study experimentally, because so many people are willing and prepared to do it, and because there are now many occupations for which this level of sleep loss is almost expected.

Partial sleep loss is considered by many researchers to be more ubiquitous in modern societies as a result of the drive for economic and social round-the-clock activity. Experimental studies suggest that it is possible for most people to maintain a fairly restricted sleeping schedule (eg down from eight hours per night to around six hours) without too many difficulties, if this is done gradually and without an abrupt shift in expected sleep patterns. Not everybody is keen on this idea, however, and there is currently considerable support for the view that many people have a nightly shortfall of sleep compared with the amount the body actually needs.

Sleep hygiene

Techniques to reinforce a sleep 'hygiene' can be useful in overcoming certain sleep-type problems, usually relating to psychological or social factors. These techniques rely on setting a regular pattern of both sleep and pre-sleep behaviours, focusing on sleep-enhancing activities, avoiding sleep inhibitors (such as caffeine or stressful situations) and preparing an environment conducive to sleep.

Zeitgebers

The term 'zeitgeber' refers to elements in the environment which exert a powerful influence on the internal body clock. This term is adapted from the German *zeit* (time) and *geber* (to give), ie 'time-giver', and encompasses many areas of daily life which provide regularity and help to adjust or 'fine-tune' the circadian clock. Natural light is particularly powerful (ie the 'natural' light and dark day), although recent changes in the way we live means that work and family life are becoming increasingly important in this respect. Examples of the major zeitgebers or daily 'regulators' are given in Fig 2 (opposite).

Sleep specifics

REM onset latency

The timing of various sleep states is an extremely important indication of normal, healthy sleep. As already explained, there are universal and predictable patterns of sleep states as indicated by changes in EEG, muscle and respiratory activity throughout the night. When this pattern breaks down, this can often can be a clue to an underlying pathological condition. REM onset latency, measured as the amount of time in minutes from the first indications of sleep to the appearance of REM sleep, can be a useful indication in this respect. Normally it takes about one-and-a-half to two hours for the first period of REM sleep to be seen in healthy adults. However, there are conditions where REM sleep onset is very fast, perhaps a matter of minutes (narcolepsy), or when REM periods occur at unusual times during the night or last longer then normal (many psychiatric conditions, including depression and schizophrenia).

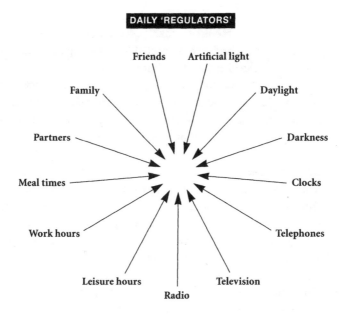

*Fig 2 **There is an enormous range of influences to encourage us to follow a regular daily routine of sleep and wake.***

Sleep efficiency

This term refers to the amount of time spent asleep after first dropping off. The idea of sleep efficiency assumes that we can quantify good sleep by its continuity. Implicit in the word 'efficiency' is the suggestion that time might be wasted here. After going to sleep, we usually expect about 10–20 minutes of wake, although most of it passes unnoticed because it is broken down into short periods, or because it is the sort of drifting in and out of sleep which is natural at the beginning and the end of a night. Similar to sleep onset latency, sleep efficiency influences our feeling of experiencing good or poor sleep. It is calculated in a number of ways, usually as a percentage or proportion of the amount of time spent in actual sleep between the first sign of sleep and getting up in the morning. The more intermittent wake during the night, the lower the sleep efficiency score.

Low sleep efficiency can be an indication of an underlying disorder of disruptive sleep, and will often leave a person feeling exhausted or unrefreshed in the morning. The cause can be both physiological, as with sleep apnoea (see opposite), or psychological, such as anxiety or depressive moods which interfere with the ability to relax into restful sleep. Excessive wakefulness during the night is problematic because it leaves us with time on our hands to ruminate over daily concerns, worry about whether we are getting enough sleep or not, and so on.

However, sleeping too soundly can indicate that we are not getting enough sleep. A certain amount of wake, particularly during the second half of the night, is normal and to be expected. Not waking up at all during the night might seem the ideal situation, but many researchers have argued that this is not the natural way to be sleeping. A high sleep efficiency score – ie little or no wake during the night – can indicate poor sleep habits or abrupt premature waking, and is usually taken as a sign of chronic insufficient sleep. So, we can expect a certain amount of waking during the night.

Sleep onset latency

This term refers to the amount of time it takes a person to fall asleep, usually from the point of turning off the light and lying down. It is a useful indication of normal sleep: we reasonably expect a sleep onset latency of around 15–30 minutes. Anything less than this may be an indication of an underlying sleep disorder (see below) or over-tiredness, ie excessive need for sleep. Longer than 30 minutes or so is also problematic, not least because of the frustration of laying in bed awake when all you want to do is sleep.

Sleep disorders

Insomnia/hypersomnia

These categories refer to a subjective account of not having the right amount of sleep. Insomnia implies not enough sleep, usually through problems in dropping off at the start of the night, or staying asleep for as long as we would like. Hypersomnia refers to an excess of sleep, ie difficulties in getting up in the morning or of avoiding sleep during the day. Both complaints have been associated with psychological factors, which may or may not be related to life events. There is also a high level of sleep complaints associated with clinical depression. Hypersomnia is more common in young depressed adults, and may help to relieve the overwhelming negative emotions during wakefulness. Conversely, insomnia is experienced by many older depressed patients, particularly the elderly or infirm.

Narcolepsy

This is a neurological disorder involving periods of excessive sleepiness during the day, often without warning. Other symptoms include paralysis of the muscles even though awake (cataplexy – see page 50), and bizarre hallucinations while falling asleep (hypnagogia – see page 50). Narcoleptics may also experience sleep paralysis, in which the body is still immobilized during the sleep/wake transition periods. Treatment is usually provided through the use of stimulants to maintain alertness during the day and to confine sleep to the night-time period.

Sleep apnoea

This is a respiratory problem in which breathing is effectively blocked for brief periods during the night, causing the individual to gasp for breath and momentarily wake themselves up in the process. The frequency of these awakenings, although brief and usually forgotten by morning, is nevertheless sufficient to interfere with the restorative qualities of sleep.

The most common reason for this involves a physical distortion of the airway and is known as obstructive sleep apnoea. Treatment for this form of apnoea involves restoring airflow using a pressurized breathing mask throughout the night or, in extreme cases, surgical reconstruction of the airway to improve breathing. A less common form of apnoea is described as central sleep apnoea. This is a neurological disorder in which the mechanisms controlling involuntary respiratory function are impaired. In rare cases, a mixture of obstructive and central sleep apnoea can be diagnosed.

The major problem in the short term is with dealing with the overwhelming sleepiness during the day caused by chronic insufficient and disturbed sleep at night. Sufferers complain of poor quality of life, although it is also argued that in extreme cases many are at more immediate risk of falling asleep inadvertently in non-stimulating environments (while driving a car, for example). For this reason, legislation is in place in certain countries to restrict driving by diagnosed sufferers subject to effective treatment, although this lacks any general consistency.

Sleep behaviours

Sleep can occasionally lead to behaviours that are distressing for both the sufferer and their family, particularly when children are involved. Excessive sleepiness and/or stress are known to be contributing factors in certain cases.

Anxiety dreams and nightmares

Perhaps the most unpleasant experience for many children and adults, the anxiety dream or nightmare is often totally unexpected and bears no resemblance to the events of the day. It emerges out of REM sleep and can nearly always be remembered, at least in part, on waking. It is often difficult to get back to sleep because of the overwhelming sense of dread and fear raised by the dream. Infrequent occurrences are to be expected and are perfectly normal. In children, they may be linked with late-night television, particularly horror films, although the link between dream content and the nightmare is often unclear.

Regular nightmares, especially with a shared theme, are worrying and they may indicate underlying psychological disturbance. Children may also develop a sense of dread about going to sleep, leading to stress and anxiety around bedtimes.

Cataplexy

This is a condition symptomatic of narcolepsy (see above), in which there is partial or complete loss of muscle control. This is often sudden and un-expected, with the individual literally falling down and being unable to move. It is known to be triggered by highly emotional or stressful states such as laughter or crying.

Hypnagogia and hynopompia

These two events occur around the ambiguous period of falling asleep and waking up, when the distinction between wake and sleep is often blurred and, even objectively, can be difficult to define. They refer to a half-sleep, dream-like state in which the mind is momentarily distracted by bizarre sen-sations or dream-like imagery and/or auditory perceptions.

It is thought that the incidence of hypnagogic (around waking up) and hypnopompic (around falling asleep) events is quite high, although fre-quency ranges from once or twice in a lifetime to many times, with some people experimenting with their own methods actually to induce them. At the time, such events can appear extremely real and convincing, if not terri-fying (see Chapter 9). These states are not dependent on being in REM sleep or normal dream states as such, but are more like flights of the imagination which occur around the brink of consciousness. It is as if the senses are engaged but are interpreting internal information as if it were real.

Night terrors

Again common in children, these are also apparent in some adults. The night terror is a perplexing event for both sufferer and parent or family. Fortunately, awakening is often incomplete and the episode is often forgotten by morning. The night terror is different in this respect from the nightmare, which usually follows a more detailed and drawn-out storyline and which almost everybody can expect from time to time. The main difference between the night terror and the nightmare is one of timing, with the night-mare stemming from REM sleep (and being more likely to occur during the second half of the night) and the night terror resulting from Stage 4 sleep, usually during the first one to two hours of sleep.

Sleep paralysis

This is an extremely frightening experience that may also include visual and auditory hallucinations. The main features are a complete or an almost complete paralysis with a clear feeling of being awake. Sleep paralysis occurs more frequently around the transition states between sleep and wake.

Sleep-walking

Sleep-walking is more common in children, although it may occur from time to time in adulthood with no prior history. Normally quite harmless, the sleep-walker is unlikely to have any recollection of the event by morning.

Other events during sleep

These can be aggravating for the sufferer, but the impact on how we feel during the day is often difficult to measure because of individual levels of tolerance and the presence, or otherwise, of related problems.

Bruxism

This is teeth grinding. It usually occurs during light sleep and can cause serious damage to the teeth. In extreme cases, dentists will fit a plastic mouthguard to be worn at night to prevent dental erosion. This is a particularly irritating condition for sleep partners, whose own sleep is often disturbed as a result.

Enuresis (bed-wetting)

Children are normally expected to be 'dry' throughout the night between two and three years of age. However, there is still a substantial proportion of children who have difficulties with this, either because it has never been completely mastered or because of relapse, possibly due to a change in home circumstances – a disturbing event for them. Bed-wetting tends to run in families, but it is not clear how far this relates to genetic factors or to family attitudes and behaviours towards toilet training. Children who wet the bed are also more likely to sleep-walk or suffer night terrors.

Leg twitching

This can be extremely irritating and disturbing for the sufferer. It tends to increase with age, but is also a complaint during some pregnancies.

Ruminations during sleep

Many people complain of being mentally active for a large part of the night. This can be because of worries spilling over into sleep. Light or disturbed sleep will leave the person feeling exhausted in the morning. It is important to go to bed with a relaxed, clear head if this is to be avoided.

Sleep talking

Also known as somniloquy, this is generally rambling and incoherent. Usually confined to NREM sleep, it may occur in combination with other behaviours such as sleep-walking. The person may attempt to respond if spoken to, although their response will not generally be consistent with the question or even make sense.

Snoring

Snoring can be an indication of a serious sleep disorder, although there is some debate on this issue. Again, partners are often the ones to suffer. A number of household remedies have been developed over the years. It is only relatively recently that the more serious implications of this behaviour have been explored.

Part 2

Sleep as a process

Chapter 4

A recipe for good sleep?

Being a 'good' sleeper is an ideal we probably all aspire to. This does not necessarily mean a heavy or indulgent sleeper, but somebody who sleeps 'efficiently' and without fuss.

What makes for good sleep? This really depends on what we are used to, what we have seen others do, and what we have come to expect. To get a sense of having slept well, most people value being able to get to sleep relatively quickly. We also expect not to wake up too often through the night, to wake up at a convenient time in the morning feeling refreshed and ready for the day, and not to need the inconvenience of sleep again during the day.

Why is it that some people find sleeping so easy, while others are left struggling? This and the following chapters address this question by looking at the issues that are involved with determining how much people sleep, and whether this is always consistent with their biological requirements.

It is probably true to say that we will all be poor sleepers at least twice in our lives: when we are babies and again towards old age. The former is not specifically our concern, whereas the latter can be a daunting prospect. There is an abundance of material providing advice and coping strategies to get through periods of difficult sleep. Common sense suggests that factors such as environment, peace of mind, diet and exercise play some part in promoting good sleep; how far these factors combine to facilitate sleep during difficult periods is perhaps the key to an understanding of a person's individual needs.

In this chapter the ability to get a 'good' night's sleep is discussed in relation to personality traits, habits, environmental conditions and hereditary factors. It seems that there is considerable responsibility on our part for setting up the right conditions for sleep, both internally and externally. The following chapters explore the 'ideal' of a consolidated period of eight hours' sleep, timed to coincide with the natural period of darkness.

Personality, peace (both as a state of mind and environmentally), practice and a genetic predisposition go a long way towards explaining why some people are better sleepers than others. Bear in mind, though, that there can be a world of difference between how much sleep we need and how much we choose to take.

Personality types and sleep

It would be misleading to think that everybody sleeps for around eight hours each night, although most people claim to (see Chapter 5). Even so, around five to ten per cent of the population sleep for unusual lengths of time (either long or short) out of choice, and seem to function well despite this.

People who regularly sleep longer than normal (about nine to ten hours per night) as a preferred choice do not describe feeling any better for it during the day than people who regularly sleep for shorter periods than normal (around five to six hours per night). The reason for this may be to do with the quality of sleep being achieved by 'short' sleepers. It seems that, even though they have a shorter night, their sleep is deep and refreshing. The additional sleep taken by 'long' sleepers is usually extra light sleep or REM sleep. So can we perhaps think of 'short' sleepers as being more 'efficient' in the way that they sleep?

The 'long' and 'short' sleepers we are talking about here are those who are convinced that this is the correct amount for them. Many people get by quite happily on these amounts, and have no difficulty in organizing their lives around this. They are simply at the extremes of a wide variation in sleep need throughout the population.

Attempts have been made to link differences in the amount and ease with which people sleep to easily defined personality traits. For example, it has often been noted that lively, out-going people appear to need less sleep than the more introverted, quieter type. A 'Type A' personality has been linked with preferred short sleep. This type of person is determined and committed in work and play, extremely active, and in constant need of stimulation. In contrast, 'Type B' personalities are generally calmer and less competitive. Most people do not fit into these extremes and fall somewhere in the middle. But it is very unlikely to be this simple – the evidence in this area is contradictory and over the years the findings on long and short sleepers have been extremely unhelpful.

For instance, both long and short sleepers have been defined as anxious, worrying types. What seems to be happening here is that people respond to psychological states and individual circumstances in different ways. Some anxious people sleep less because their worries interfere with sleep, whereas others sleep more, perhaps because their worries interfere with their wake time and sleep may offer a comforting release from the pressures of the day. This tends to be particularly true for some teenagers, who are prone to dark moods and prefer to lie in bed for most of the day. So, there are a number of problems with equating 'type' of person to how much they sleep. Some people just need unusual amounts of sleep for physiological reasons, and this is perfectly normal given the diversity of normal populations. Others may be responding to circumstances in their life, but more on this later.

It may be that short sleep reflects choices in lifestyle which might otherwise not be achievable on long sleep, such as extensive work or leisure commitments. For that reason, it is often difficult to separate 'natural' short sleepers from those who arrive at this pattern through self-discipline alone. However, these descriptions can be very judgemental, in favour of the 'high-achieving' short sleeper. They represent stereotypes, reinforcing the idea that sleep patterns – like other excesses such as over-eating, heavy drinking and over-spending – can say something very definite about the type of person you are. It seems that we are far more tolerant, even admiring, of short sleepers, who are merely 'burning the candle at both ends' to get things done.

This is consistent with the compulsive hard worker, who doesn't seem to need much sleep at all. This person may also have strong views on sleep, and be quick to let people know. Thomas Edison managed with very little sleep. So did Napoleon, Winston Churchill and Margaret Thatcher, all renowned for strong leadership skills and high achievement. Edison was, in fact, quite outspoken on this issue, believing that a great deal of sleep was merely habit and imitation, serving no real physical purpose. Contrast this with the long sleeper who likes to get to bed way before midnight and stay there for nine or even ten hours. While the short sleeper is viewed as dynamic and active, living life to the full, the long sleeper is seen as self-indulgent, lazy, plodding and lacking in drive. The association between oversleeping and laziness or slothfulness has been around for some time, and is typically described as an

A brief distraction: 'personality'

Although not all advocates of personality measures view the individual as a set of stable, measurable traits or types, there has been tremendous support for the idea of personality 'types', filtering down to the popular level through magazine 'quizzes' and the like. This approach offers a relatively simple means of collecting information about differences between individuals on a large scale. Very often this involves asking people about their likes and dislikes; their usual patterns of social interaction; whether they avoid or encourage the company of others; and how they would respond to a series of hypothetical situations, from speaking in public to spending time on their own. The aim in all this is to get some idea of what drives people to behave in the way that they do and how this determines lifestyles. Most personality scales assume that there are a number of universal traits which, although unique in combination for each individual, offers some insight into what makes a person the way they are.

However, broad generalizations and ideas implicit about people of a particular personality 'type' can actually taint perceptions and influence the way we respond to each other. Often, this is based on stereotypical assumptions. Nor is it obvious how far personality helps to explain response to individual circumstances. When do we begin to take on the characteristics of a particular personality type due to the experience of life events? Are we tied to a personality trait, such as introversion, throughout our life?

undesirable habit and one which does not bode well for the future: 'Love not sleep, lest thou come to poverty' (Proverbs 20:13).

However, it is extremely difficult to separate long and short sleepers who have a genuine difference in sleep need from people who follow these extremes due to pressing economic, social or psychological circumstances. It could be that personality factors are linked with sleep need, but it is equally likely that they will also determine occupational and social activities, factors that inevitably influence how sleepy we feel at the end of the day.

Practice

Can successful sleep habits be learned through practice? It seems that for young, healthy adults the ability to sleep well is fairly stable, barring obvious upset. By middle age, however, most people's sleep requirement begins to change. EEG studies show that from around this age there is a gradual reduction in deep sleep (Stages 3 and 4) and that getting to sleep can be more problematic for many people.

The idea that we can train ourselves or practise to be good sleepers by following a few simple guidelines has widespread appeal. This is often referred to as sleep 'hygiene' and is a first line of attack for dealing with emerging difficulties. The emphasis in this self-help approach is on developing a good routine, and often this means following a few simple guidelines such as those presented in Table 1 (overleaf).

Exercise is definitely not a good idea shortly before going to bed. Rather than wearing you out, it can have the opposite effect of stimulating you, ready for action. Hot baths, on the other hand, encourage physical and mental relaxation and really do encourage deeper sleep, at least in the early part of the night. We should also avoid watching dramatic television programmes or films which are likely to be emotionally disturbing.

But can we really 'learn' how to sleep? Certainly, worrying about sleep is likely to be very important in reinforcing an already difficult situation. We can also learn, through practice and experience, when it is a good time for us to sleep, and when we should just give it up (there is more on this in Chapter 6). Through getting to know our own needs, it is possible to learn to create the conditions conducive to sleep.

But whether or not we can learn to sleep at will is open to debate. This would mean being able to sleep even when we don't really need to. Bizarrely, this was tried with rats in the mid-1970s[1]. The experiment relied on a technique known as 'behavioural conditioning', whereby a system of rewards and punishments are used to reinforce certain behaviours. In this case, the experimenters wished to know if it were possible for rats to fall asleep 'at will'. In order to do this, it was necessary to arouse the rats' interest in performing the required behaviour. This was achieved by rewarding the rats with food immediately following each period of spontaneous sleep, thereby establishing a positive association between sleep and reward. In this way, the rats were encouraged to expect more food each time they were able to sleep, ie they were literally taught to 'sleep' for food. And this was achieved with some success: as the rats gradually made the connection between sleep and food, they spent more and more of their time in 'sleep-like' postures, making beds, closing their eyes and curling up. However, despite this obvious will to sleep, the rats were merely faking it and none of them was able actually to fall asleep unless they genuinely needed it.

In humans, it often takes some time to adapt to unusual circumstances. Sleeping in the unfamiliar surroundings of a sleep laboratory can take at least one and perhaps more nights to settle down, although this is not always practicable due to costs. Many laboratories now use portable monitoring equipment, which enables the patient or volunteer to remain in their own home during all-night sleep recordings and so achieve a more realistic picture of their regular sleep patterns.

Falling asleep can be an extremely anxious time, with problems soon escalating out of control. Sleeping pills have their uses in the short term, because the individual can have confidence in their effectiveness and anxiety about falling to sleep unaided is reduced – so much so, that on occasion people have been found to sleep better after taking a decoy pill, or 'placebo', which has no known therapeutic action.

Table 1 **Recommendations for enhancing sleep 'hygiene'.**

DO
• Keep to roughly the same bedtime every night.
• Maintain a predictable daily pattern of activity.
• Avoid exercise in the early evening.
• Practice relaxation techniques (mental and physical) before going to bed.
• Whenever possible, deal with troubling issues rather than putting them off for the next day.
• Associate the bedroom with sleep – not television, reading, etc.

DO NOT
• Worry about the effects of not getting enough sleep: we need less as we get older anyway and we are able to put even a small amount of sleep to good use.
• Nap during the day to supplement poor sleep at night. This will only set up a vicious circle which it is hard to break out of.
• Stay in bed later in the morning to make up for a difficult night. Again, this will only set up bad habits.
• Spend too long in bed if you cannot get to sleep. Give it about half an hour and then get up and do something else until you feel sleepy again.
• Drink tea or coffee from the early evening onwards, as this is likely to interfere with sleep.
• Drink excessive amounts of alcohol. In the short term it may help you fall asleep, but there is more chance of being wide awake in the middle of the night.

Peace of mind

Sleep difficulties are often responses to a more basic problem, such as depression or anxiety, which may be short-lived. During severe depression, difficulty in getting off to sleep, lengthy periods of wake during the night, and waking up too early in the morning are frequent complaints. The other extreme, oversleeping, is also normal and is again dependent on individual response to negative situations.

In the 1970s and 1980s there was a great deal of enthusiasm for sleep deprivation as a non-invasive treatment for mood disorders, following the discovery of an improvement in mood for depressed patients who were encouraged to stay up all night without sleep. This was tried out with in-patients on psychiatric wards who had previously failed to respond to the usual drug or behavioural treatments. In around 60 per cent of all reported cases, the depressed mood was lifted towards the end of the night. Unfortunately, this effect was short-lived as most patients relapse into their original mood state following a single episode of sleep. Nevertheless, the link between sleep (particularly REM sleep) and mood has fuelled debate over the importance of dreaming for emotional well-being (see Chapter 12).

The association between sleep and mood is intriguing: waking up in a bad mood is almost always put down to not looking forward to the day's events, rather than its being a natural part of the sleep process. Yet, not sleeping often has the opposite effect by raising mood. These changes can be quite noticeable in sleep-deprivation experiments: volunteers become less inhibited and will joke, laugh and generally be more mischievous as time goes by.

Insomnia

Problems with sleep that may have been initiated by a difficult period will sometimes develop into a more long-term issue, reinforced by each experience of poor sleep. Anxiety about going to bed and expectations of poor sleep combine to ensure repeated failures. So, what can be done when it is not always possible to leave behind the events of the day and relax into undisturbed sleep?

Our understanding of the process of actually falling asleep is far from complete. Under normal conditions, sleep relies simply on everything falling into place at the same time: a sleepy body, a willing mind, and a peaceful, comfortable environment. When all goes well, we have no real sense of the fragility of this process. When it does not, things can quickly spiral out of control.

Self-diagnosed insomnia is widespread. Although the use of sleeping pills is a popular method for treating insomnia, particularly in the elderly, it is not generally suitable for long-term use because of the difficulty of shaking off the effects the next morning and the risk of dependency over time. Similarly, many insomniacs use alcohol to help with sleep. This is also not to be recommended because, although alcohol can have quite a strong sedative effect, it tends to interfere with the normal pattern of sleep 'stages' across the night, which in turn reduces the overall subjective quality of the night's sleep.

People who complain of insomnia often display a wide variety of symptoms, suggesting that a tolerance for getting by with less sleep is perhaps equally as important as more objective measures of actual sleep in identifying a problem. Typical complaints include difficulty with getting off to sleep (up to hours on end), waking through the night, waking up too early, or waking up feeling dreadful and still in need of sleep by morning.

Often, the condition of sleeplessness is only temporary and can be linked with a specific unsettling event, such as a marriage break-up or loss of work. In these cases, the reasons for not being able to sleep are clearly to do with the worry and anxiety of that particular set of circumstances. There is every chance that when things improve and become more settled emotionally, normal sleep will resume. Most people need to go to bed feeling mentally relaxed and reasonably trouble free in order to sleep peacefully. When this is not possible, and the mind becomes fixated on troubles or worries, then the body's drive for sleep is easily overridden. As the hours tick by, the urgency for sleep and worries about getting through the next day make things worse, and anxiety levels escalate.

Not all insomnia is event-related but may be part of a more ongoing, general problem. There may be a physiological explanation, in terms of the brain mechanisms responsible for the transition between wake and sleep, although this is often difficult to establish because of the interdependence between physiological and psychological factors. The effect of not being able to sleep freely will almost inevitably lead to anxiety and stress, which may reinforce the situation through expectations of sleep difficulties, perhaps even after the original problem has been settled. This builds up into a cycle of reinforcement, whereby the insomniac expects to have difficulties and is not optimistic about going to bed. These negative beliefs and anxieties play on the mind after lights out and make falling to sleep extremely difficult, hence justifying and reinforcing the original expectations.

A number of treatments aimed at breaking into this cycle have been successful by homing in on the insomniac's worries about not getting enough sleep. One of the biggest concerns among insomniacs is that they are not getting 'normal' sleep and that they must in some way, perhaps physically, be suffering as a result. These fears can place unrealistic demands on a system that may not, in the present circumstances, need or be able to achieve this amount of sleep. Many treatment programmes address these issues directly, with a view to reducing the concern for more sleep.

A novel approach to this was adopted recently in the Netherlands, where researchers broadcast a newly devised treatment programme over an eight-week run of national television and radio programmes[2]. These attracted an initial audience of over 200,000 viewers, over 10 per cent of whom went on to 'register' as participants and to receive additional literature (sleep diaries, guide books, etc) to supplement the broadcast information. Many of the group had suffered long-term difficulties, with over half reporting symptoms dating back over ten years. A proportion of those taking part were monitored in order to assess the overall effectiveness of the programme.

One of the main aims of the treatment was to get away from the idea of using sleeping pills in cases of chronic insomnia. Instead, the schedule of programmes was based around:
• Educating the individual about 'normal' sleep.
• Emphasizing the importance of establishing a regular routine and taking personal control of this.
• Helping with mental and physical relaxation.

An important feature of this involved keeping detailed records of all periods of sleep and wake activity, in order to encourage participants to look for areas of their waking life which might help towards explaining their current sleep difficulties. One of the strengths in this method is the empowering of the individual with responsibility for their own treatment, rather than handing it over to a pharmacological remedy. The aim is that as the insomniac becomes more knowledgeable about sleep as a whole, they are able to put their own problems into a more realistic perspective. The programme addressed many of the common-sense ideas about sleep, and participants were given detailed information concerning current theories about why we sleep, the wide variations in normal behaviour, and the effects of psychological stress on sleep. Essentially, participants were equipped with a better understanding of what was happening to them.

The programme proved to be effective for many of those who completed the eight-week course. Over 40 per cent who had previously used sleeping pills no longer relied on them. Many also reported not taking as long to fall asleep at night, and sleeping longer through the night. What was particularly encouraging was that these positive effects of the programme were still being reported five months later.

Although on the face of it this treatment was extremely effective, it is important to note that these were not medically diagnosed insomniacs, and positive effects were measured subjectively by the volunteers themselves. There was also very little direct professional screening of the pre- or post-treatment levels of sleep difficulty. Yet despite these limitations, the treatment programme was considered a success. The advantage in locating control firmly with the individual is that the individual was able to deal directly with the problem, whereas a sleeping pill simply knocks one out. Getting one good night's sleep with a pill is unlikely to improve your chances of a repeat performance on the next night, and it may even make things worse.

Peace and quiet

Living next door to a busy road with constant traffic noise throughout the night can be a daunting prospect for many people. This is likely to be a pressing problem for the future, if traffic density and night transportation continue to escalate at their present rate. Many government agencies are willing to fund households living near roads with heavy traffic flow for part of the cost of double-glazing their windows, as an attempt to insulate them from the 'pollution' of external noise. Pressure groups have been influential in highlighting the detrimental effects of noise on sleep. Of course, many people survive living next to busy motorways, railways and airports, and anecdotal reports suggest that some people are completely oblivious to this after a while. But not everybody is willing to take the risk: house prices are noticeably cheaper next to major airports, and proposals for additional airports or even runways on existing sites are objected to vociferously.

In the laboratory, considerable effort has gone into studying the effects of regular and loud external noise on the quality and continuity of sleep. A recent Japanese study monitored the effects on over 3,000 women of living next to a road with heavy night-time traffic[3]. As you might expect, sleep problems (mainly insomnia) were substantially greater for those women living closest to the road. However, studies looking at the effect of being exposed to noise for the first time (similar to moving into a new house) have shown that over a period of time it is possible for some people to become inured to the familiar noise outside their bedroom window. Novelty is the key here – you do not become tolerant to noise in general, but to you own particular setting, whether that includes trains, aeroplanes or motorway traffic. In fact, once this has happened, an unusually 'peaceful' environment, such as a trip to the country for a city-dweller, can have the paradoxical effect of being too quiet for the first night or two.

It seems that we are not entirely oblivious, however. A Dutch study recently investigated the effectiveness of using 'double' glazing to prevent disturbance from heavy traffic noise[4]. This was a particularly interesting study, in that it was shown that although volunteers did not wake up to every passing heavy vehicle, they still responded to it with an increase in heart rate. This was the case even following a series of nights which allowed volunteers to become familiar with the noise. Apparently we can monitor noise on some level without actually waking up. Some people are more sensitive to this than others.

There are other environmental factors, such as daylight hours and temperature, which are likely to have an effect on sleep. Sleep duration and sleep quality have a strong seasonal component, with many people finding they sleep longer in the winter than the summer months. This also has strong associations with mood, and at its most extreme is classified as a clinical disorder: Seasonal Affective Disorder (SAD), more commonly known as 'winter blues'. Differences between winter and summer sleep patterns are more pronounced for populations living in the northern hemisphere compared with those in equatorial regions, suggesting that the more pronounced changes in climactic conditions are indeed a factor.

People with SAD experience a range of symptoms in association with sleep changes. These include negative moods, change in appetite and weight (increase or loss), lack of energy, and loss of enthusiasm for social activities. Many sufferers find symptoms improve in the spring, only to return again the following winter. Seasonal differences in hours of natural sunlight have been thought to be in part responsible for this syndrome, a theory supported by the positive effect of substituting daily doses of strong artificial light during the winter months (phototherapy). During treatment, patients sit in front of a powerful 'lightbox', often in their own home. The mechanisms for enhancing mood with this approach are unclear, although developments in this area have accelerated recently owing to public and scientific interest. There is also considerable enthusiasm for light treatment in the areas of shift-work and jet lag, because of its potential for rescheduling sleep.

In order to sleep comfortably, most of us are able to tolerate only a very narrow 'window' of temperature settings: the ambient surroundings should be neither too hot nor too cold. The second condition is easier to deal with by wearing more clothes or putting an extra duvet on the bed. Overheating is more difficult and in the summer months there is often a real battle to sleep.

Genetic predisposition

There has been considerable interest in the possibility of hereditary traits in sleep behaviours. This would help to account for the vast range in sleep patterns observed in the population. The obvious approach is to ask whether people in the same family sleep for similar lengths of time. Unfortunately, with regard to sleep behaviours it can be difficult to know how much of this is physiological, when family members experience the same 'training' through years of living together.

Most of the evidence in this area stems from studies of the sleeping patterns of adult twins. For example, in Finland in the 1970s, all adult twins of the same sex were traced through birth registration documents and invited to take part in a study of genetic influences on sleep patterns; almost 7,000 agreed[5]. One-third of the twin pairs were 'identical' (monozygotic), with the remainder being 'non-identical' (dizygotic). Volunteers gave detailed responses to questionnaires about their lifestyles, including normal sleep patterns, satisfaction, difficulties, etc. In analysing the data, researchers found a clear positive indication that sleep habits are indeed shared by the same family members; twin brothers and sisters in the study were more likely to have similar sleep patterns than you would expect by chance from two people of the same age and sex. With this large group of participants, it was only when they reached their early twenties, and then just for men, that circumstances forced twins living apart to follow quite different sleep patterns.

Closer studies of EEG sleep recordings in twins have also shown that, whether living together or not, twins are similar in how much time they spend getting to sleep, their likelihood of waking up during the night, and how much Stage 3, 4 and REM sleep they get. These findings are even stronger in the case of identical twins.

Do sleep preferences run in the family? It seems so, and this is the case even when they no longer live together. However, it is often difficult to tease apart environmental and social factors from the influence of genetic make-up, which appears to be easily overwhelmed. But if you were able to take away the entire range of social factors, lifestyles, anxieties, environmental conditions, personal habits, etc, then it seems probable that what would be left is a strong, genetically determined basis for how much we sleep. It is debatable just how many people can not only recognize their physiological sleep needs but also achieve these in the face of a wide range of competing distractions.

A recipe for good sleep?

An important move towards achieving a good night's sleep involves getting to know just how much you normally sleep, whether there are certain periods or conditions when it is most satisfying, and which times during the day or night are perhaps most troublesome.

The best way to do this is to record sleep patterns over a series of days or even weeks. Usually this needs to be around one to two weeks to be of any use. This involves making up a simple diary of sleep patterns; a typical sleep 'diary' is shown in Fig 3 (opposite). It is then possible to chart the various factors, such as bedtimes, sleep duration, feeling refreshed in the morning, sleep quality, etc against each other. More complex versions can also include mood and sleepiness states throughout the day, or work or social patterns.

By making a systematic recording in this way, it often transpires that people who think they are getting a standard eight hours sleep per night are quite surprised to find that they do in fact sleep much closer to seven hours per night, or even less. We also have a short memory for the benefits of a good night's sleep, and by recording additional information about sleep quality and early-morning feelings a diary such as this can help establish a link between feeling good and well timed sleep.

Short-term factors

Clearly, there are a number of factors which explain differences in sleep habits, some of which are more stable than others. In addition to these

SLEEP DIARY

This diary is to be used to record sleep patterns for a minimum of seven days. Shade the appropriate squares according to the key below to indicate how long you sleep for each night. Keep the diary next to your bedside and fill it in first thing in the morning before you get up. You should also record any sleep taken during the day.

Key to shading ☐ Awake   ■ Asleep   ☒ In bed but awake

DAY 1

8am 10am noon 2pm 4pm 6pm 8pm 10pm midnight 2am 4am 6am

How well did you sleep last night?   Excellent   Good   Quite poor   Very poor
                                           ○   ○   ○   ○

How sleepy do you feel right now?   Extremely   Quite   Hardly   Not at all
                                           ○   ○   ○   ○

DAY 2

8am 10am noon 2pm 4pm 6pm 8pm 10pm midnight 2am 4am 6am

How well did you sleep last night?   Excellent   Good   Quite poor   Very poor
                                           ○   ○   ○   ○

How sleepy do you feel right now?   Extremely   Quite   Hardly   Not at all
                                           ○   ○   ○   ○

DAY 3

8am 10am noon 2pm 4pm 6pm 8pm 10pm midnight 2am 4am 6am

How well did you sleep last night?   Excellent   Good   Quite poor   Very poor
                                           ○   ○   ○   ○

How sleepy do you feel right now?   Extremely   Quite   Hardly   Not at all
                                           ○   ○   ○   ○

Now continue on another sheet for days 4–7

Fig 3 **A sleep diary, kept long term, can help reveal strong patterns in sleep behaviours.**

variables, in the short term we often knowingly or unwittingly indulge in substances which interfere with how well we sleep.

Food has for a long time been considered a potential source of nightmares and disturbance, and heavy lunches are often blamed for excessive sleepiness. The sedating properties of alcohol are well known and provide readily available relief for late-night insomniacs. We also rely on caffeine, often in conjunction with cigarettes, as one of the most convenient aids to avoiding sleep. Yet all these substances impact on sleep quality to some extent.

In 1979 researchers from Oxford University looked at the long-term effects of smoking and drinking alcohol on sleep duration and quality[6]. Over 1,500 people from small villages in Oxfordshire volunteered to provide details of their normal smoking, drinking and sleeping patterns. These details were analysed to look for specific connections between differences in sleep patterns for people who regularly smoked and drank alcohol and those who didn't. The findings were quite striking – non-smokers and teetotallers slept for an average of an extra half hour each night. While non-smokers normally slept for about seven-and-a-half hours each night, smokers were getting only seven hours, with those smoking over 40 cigarettes a day sleeping half an hour less than this. A similar pattern was true for alcohol use. Teetotallers slept for an average of seven-and-a-half hours compared with only six-and-a-half for heavy drinkers (over nine units of alcohol per night).

Perhaps surprisingly, though, when asked to assess their sleep in terms of quality, smokers did not judge it to be of poorer quality than non-smokers. This may have been a little misleading, for a number of reasons. Subjective measures do not deal in absolutes, but rely on individuals making relative assessments compared with how they usually feel. What is considered 'normal' for one group may be unusual for another. For example, after years of drinking alcohol every night, a person might consider a single trip to the bathroom in the middle of the night quite normal, and rate their sleep as relatively undisturbed, ie 'good'. In contrast, somebody who is not used to this might consider waking up in the middle of the night due to a full bladder somewhat unusual and describe this as a 'disturbed' night's sleep.

There is also a tendency to underestimate the impact of alcohol on sleep, possibly because we are misled by the fact that it actually induces sleepiness in the short term and for that reason is often used as a sleep aid. And yet in objective studies, it is clear that alcohol has undesirable effects on sleep.

• After drinking even a moderate amount of alcohol, sleep tends to be heavier in the early part of the night, meaning that the individual is more difficult to rouse than usual. REM sleep is delayed or reduced relative to sober sleep.

• Alcohol also affects respiratory function, which, because sleep is inordinately deep in the early part of the night, increases the risk of vomit inhalation during sleep.

• Sleep continuity is also disturbed throughout the second half of the night.

The more unpleasant symptoms of a 'hangover' may appear by this stage. Disturbance through getting up and going to the bathroom is increased.
• Aside from the more obvious after-effects of alcohol (dehydration, sickness, headaches), there may be a direct effect on mood ('booze blues') following the disruption of REM sleep.

Alcohol can also have a different effect depending on how sleepy we are at the time we drink it, with the most serious problems occurring in combination with acute sleep deprivation. Even afternoon alcohol intake can often have a stronger effect on alertness simply because it coincides with a natural dip in arousal at around this time. Afternoon drinking can also have a profound negative effect on the quality of sleep the same night, leading to more superficial sleep and waking towards the second half of the night.

In young adults, smoking is associated with a similar reduction in sleep. Twenty per cent of a recent sample of 14-year-olds from English secondary schools admitted smoking regularly. They were more likely to go to bed late and sleep less than non-smoking teenagers from the same group. There are obviously many factors involved here, and it may be that whatever draws young adults to smoking also provides a disincentive for them to sleep (peer pressure, urgency to 'grow up', etc), rather than the smoking itself interfering with the physical ability to sleep.

Many people are aware of feeling drowsy in the early afternoon but take countermeasures such as coffee, fresh air, or walking about to avoid actually falling to sleep. It is often felt that the reason for this afternoon 'dip' is in some way connected with eating over the lunchtime period. And yet, if you go without lunch the sleepiness will still appear at around the same time. What seems to be happening here is that the circadian effect leading to afternoon sleepiness is further enhanced by large, high-fat meals taken at around the same time. Meals of similar nutritional quality but taken in a liquid form do not have such a strong effect, so bulk may be an important factor here. A high-carbohydrate meal at lunchtime will not necessarily make you sleep faster – but it seems that if you do decide to take a nap then you are likely to sleep longer than on an empty stomach. The mechanisms to explain this are unclear. If it is important to stay awake and be on top form throughout the afternoon, then rather than skip lunch, a light snack and no alcohol is perhaps the best option.

Achieving a balance

It should now be clear that the message of this chapter is that in order to be 'good' sleepers we need to reach a delicate balance between a wide range of factors – physiological, environmental and social – which can only be achieved through getting to know what is right for our own unique set of circumstances.

Chapter 5
How much sleep do we need?

Sources of general health advice such as popular magazines and family medical books often suggest that the optimum amount of sleep each night for a healthy adult is somewhere in the region of seven to eight hours. The origins of this belief lie somewhere between the relatively recent scheduling of organized economic behaviour and observations *en masse* of personal experience.

Although variation in sleep patterns across the whole population is huge, the ideal of the 'eight-hour sleep' has strong currency in today's society. Equally important is the belief that we should get all this sleep in one block during the night, rather than spread across the day. But is this really the ideal way to sleep?

There are a number of reasons for asking these questions. Firstly, despite the spectacular efforts of Randy Gardner, John Hart and Peter Tripp (see Chapter 1), sleep is still generally understood to perform an essential function, the benefits of which can be found in our ability to cope with the rigours of daily life. This implies that less than adequate sleep at night will lead to an inevitable reduction in our ability to perform tasks that are both physically and mentally demanding, including the ability to operate machinery, to drive, to concentrate over long periods, to learn, to remember and even to interact socially. Without such concerns, the amount of sleep an individual takes would be left largely to personal choice. Instead, interest in sleep has accumulated at such a pace that many occupational, industrial, government, health and even legal agencies now claim a legitimate interest in trends in sleep behaviour throughout the general population.

'America has a sleep debt and in our opinion it is every bit as important as the national debt'. This remark was made on behalf of the USA-based National Commission on Sleep Disorders in 1993 and gives an indication of the strength of feeling for the whole issue of sleep in today's society. The implication here is that sleep loss is a serious problem for many Americans, who face adverse effects on health, accident rates, productivity and educational achievement. These issues are discussed in more depth in Chapter 14. But first, there are a number of questions which are fundamental to this debate, and these are discussed in this chapter.

How much do we sleep?

It is extremely difficult to know just how much people actually sleep. The assumption that most people sleep for around eight hours is based on population studies that involved simply asking people how much they slept. There are a number of problems with this approach.

Firstly, it relies on people being accurate in their estimations. The idea of eight hours' sleep being normal has been around for so long now that it may be automatic to quote this amount without thinking. After all, without a genuine concern for one's own sleep patterns, it is not usual to examine them in any great depth. Sleep duration also fluctuates depending on current circumstances. The differences between weekday and weekend sleep can amount to one or two hours for many people. These differences are lost when we try to pin people down to a single estimate of how much they sleep. This is complicated further by the fact that people are often reluctant to appear different. The alternative, however – to provide objective monitoring using equipment and laboratory staff – is costly and labour intensive, and is usually limited to hundreds rather than thousands of participants.

Despite these difficulties, surveys using telephone interviews or postal questionnaires have provided valuable data on normal, in-the-home, adult sleep patterns. The more substantial of these endorse the idea that most people aim for seven to eight hours' sleep each night, and that this is a trend which establishes towards the teenage years. But why isn't this the same for everybody, and what happens when things go wrong?

What are the health risks associated with sleep length?

In the 1960s and early 1970s, a series of reports suggested that there might be a critical link between how much we sleep at night and the risk of serious health problems.

In 1967, the American Cancer Society canvassed information on lifestyle and habits (including sleep) from over one million Americans, with a view to isolating those factors contributing to the onset of cancer[1]. This survey was to provide an important insight into the sleeping patterns of the average American. Respondents, all drawn from friends, family and neighbours of society members, were asked to complete a detailed questionnaire at the onset of the study, and then again six years later. The survey dealt with all areas of normal, daily activity including diet, cigarette smoking, alcohol consumption and drug use, but also covered details of normal sleep duration, including in particular the question ' How many hours of sleep do you usually get a night?' As might be expected, the average sleep duration was found to be between seven and eight hours per night. Perhaps more importantly, though, initial analysis showed that respondents who claimed to sleep for relatively short (less than four hours) or long (more than nine hours) periods at night were far more likely to have died before the six-year follow-up. Cause of death for excessive sleep lengths (greater than ten hours per night) was linked with an increase in stroke and heart disease.

A similar finding was made in a large Californian survey at around the same time, in which nearly 7,000 residents of Alameda County took part[2]. Respondents on this occasion were all in their middle age and chosen at random from census records. The first screening took place in 1965 and involved completing a lengthy questionnaire. Again, the topics covered many general aspects of health and lifestyle, including specific questions on length and quality of sleep. From this data it was clear that, on average, most respondents slept between seven and nine hours each night. This was by no means the case for all respondents, though, as the range of sleep duration covered anything from around four hours each night to more than ten hours.

Nine years later, in 1974, a follow-up survey was conducted to examine relationships between lifestyles and health. Almost 400 of the original respondents had died during the intervening period. Attention was drawn to the fact that men and women who slept for less than four hours or more than nine hours were almost twice as likely to have died in the interim period than those sleeping for eight hours at night. Overall, seven-and-a-half to eight hours' sleep each night was associated with proportionately fewer cases of cancer, stroke and heart disease. Not only that, but respondents' health before the 1965 survey could not account for these findings, ie ill-health did not seem to be the reason why some of the sample had adopted unusual and extreme sleep patterns.

Both surveys suggested an important association between sleep and health, reinforcing the idea that we should all be aiming for eight hours' sleep at night. The reasons for this apparent increase in health risk following deviations from the eight-hour sleep remain unclear, although it seems likely that the factors which determine unusual patterns of sleep, such as work or social habits, are important considerations. We also need to put things in proportion, as the link between sleep duration and mortality highlighted in these studies may not be a causal one, and as a 'risk' factor, sleep duration was nowhere near as important as smoking, excessive alcohol, diet or lack of exercise.

Sleep duration in itself need not necessarily lead to poor health, but may be an indication that something else is going on. For example, a recent survey examined the relationships between diet, lifestyle (including sleeping patterns) and health in almost 4,000 Dutch nationals[3]. It was found that people who slept for less than seven hours at night tended to follow a high-fat diet, drank high levels of alcohol and smoked. Obviously this is not the full picture, but it is a reminder that the decision to sleep is taken as part of a much wider context than physiology alone.

What are the major influences on sleep patterns?

On an intuitive level, many of us have first-hand experience of sleep disturbance in the short-term, perhaps over a series of particularly late nights due to work or social commitments, and may have felt unable to function as normal. Very often, the genuine effects of losing sleep are clouded by the circumstances leading up to it, and our perception of discomfort will depend largely on our willingness to go without sleep.

The decision to sleep is influenced by a wide range of physiological, psychological, environmental and social factors, some of which are illustrated in Fig 4. The influence of a particular factor will vary in intensity over time. This can act in both directions. So, for example, in a nightclub at 2am the body might need sleep, but it is unlikely that this will happen because of the arousing effect of noise, and social and psychological stimulation. At the other extreme, many people find long, monotonous car or coach journeys too boring to stay awake for and can easily doze into light sleep for much of the journey. This is because, in the absence of social or environmental stimulation, there is little resistance to the physiological factors urging us to sleep (such as time of day), even though these may be only moderate to low in intensity at that time. In these circumstances, we could say that the decision to sleep is negotiable and will depend on our willingness to resist. This is not to say that sleep can always be avoided by sheer force of will, and it would be extremely naïve, and often dangerous, to expect this to be the case.

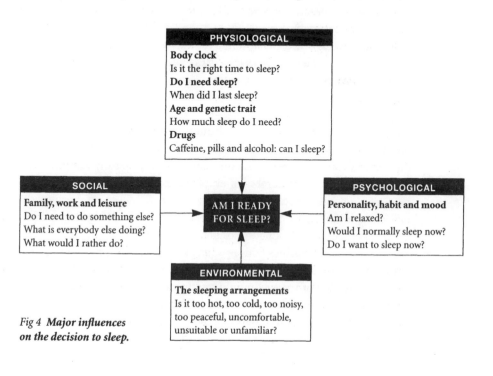

Fig 4 Major influences on the decision to sleep.

Normally we are able to balance the needs of the body with the demands of family, friends and work. We facilitate this by setting aside regular periods for sleep in quiet, dark and relaxing areas of the home. Occasionally, this balance is upset as a particular factor assumes dominance over other areas, and often at the expense of hours available for sleep.

The importance of circadian and external factors has already been touched on in describing fundamental areas of basic sleep research. Sleep patterns have also been linked with genes, psychology, environmental conditions and force of habit. However, it is arguably social factors that lead to the most ongoing disruption in sleep patterns, and which are increasingly at odds with the internal, physiological drive for sleep.

There is compelling evidence to suggest that many individuals are able to cope with relatively short periods of sleep without detrimental effects. At the other extreme, some people find that eight hours' sleep is simply not enough and that they are only fully refreshed if they are able to sleep closer to nine or even ten hours each night. In terms of waking effectiveness, people sleeping at the extreme of sleep patterns do not generally show consistent differences in their alertness or efficiency when performing tasks during the day. For example, the short sleeper does not seem to have an advantage in terms of alertness or efficiency, as is the general perception. The long sleeper simply takes a bit longer at night to reach this level. What is important is to be able to recognize when the amount of sleep we take at night is incompatible with our physical needs.

One way to approach this question is to look at the various reasons which crop up from time to time to prevent us from sleeping perhaps as much as we would like. In that sense, the flexibility of the human sleep system in being able to cope with these changes is in many ways more important than the concept of an absolute sleep requirement.

Sleep in context: zeitgebers

The amount we sleep is very much a question of how far our decision to sleep coincides with other things going on in our lives. Chapter 1 introduced the idea of a social zeitgeber as an important 'regulator' of daily patterns. This term describes the vast number of events in and around the world which regulate our behaviours to a daily, weekly and sometimes yearly schedule. For many people the day's events are, by and large, orderly and predictable. With the occasional exception, bedtimes and waketimes are reasonably stable across the weeks. We achieve this by organizing our lives around the dominant zeitgebers at the time. These will include natural factors (such as the rising and setting of the sun and fluctuations in temperature) and social factors (work hours, meal times and leisure times). Without such reminders, we are left pretty much to the timing of our own internal clock to decide when to be active and when to be asleep. Although remarkably accurate, the coincidence with the external 'day' is not guaranteed. Zeitgebers help to 'fine-tune' our natural rhythms to a pattern in keeping with our daily lives.

Zeitgebers which are known to have a powerful influence on sleep patterns include:
• Work.
• Family life, especially partner.
• Lifestyles, use of caffeine, alcohol, drugs or tobacco.
• Environment.

Our decision to sleep and for how long is determined largely by the combined influences of these factors, as well as age, state of mind, and a physiological sleep need. Although we are usually able to balance the interests of both the body and the mind, occasionally things can go wrong.

Any disruption to the regulating features of our day is likely to have a knock-on effect on sleep patterns. Major changes, such as a new house or change of job, can take some adjustment. Conflict arises where we are unable to satisfy the body's requirements for sleep because of the distraction of particularly powerful zeitgebers in our social world.

This can sometimes be an abrupt change in circumstances, through bereavement or loss of job, for example. Even when disruption is anticipated, as with the arrival of a new baby, there is very little that parents can do to prepare themselves for the forced change in their sleep habits. Not all change is for the worse, however. With the right motivation, even major changes in sleep patterns can be tolerated well in the short term. The critical factors tend to be length of disruption, ease of adaptation and frame of mind.

What happens when things go wrong?

The factors that interfere with getting a good night's sleep include:

Work

Sleep disturbances are often understood to give a good indication of the early signs of physical and mental problems during periods of potential stress. This has been highlighted in many large-scale studies of sleep behaviours, where a close link has been found with reduced or poor-quality sleep and the presence of psychological or social difficulties. For this reason, a number of researchers have concentrated on the effects of major upheaval on patterns of sleep. As governments have a vested interest in national health, many of them have a policy of regular monitoring by homing in on a cross-section of the population selected to cover a broad range of ages and occupational groups. This has allowed governments to take a 'snapshot' of the population at regular intervals and to relate findings concerning health and lifestyle to the prevailing economic and social conditions. This has been a particularly useful approach in assessing the long-term effects of the introduction of social policies concerning health, welfare or education, for example. It can also give some insight into the effects of a more general economic change.

Financial stability is one of the major concerns for any individual. The threat of unemployment brings with it doubts about where we will be living and the quality of life to be expected over an indefinite period. Very few people would be untroubled by this situation, particularly if they have come to expect regular, steady employment. The effects of unemployment, in both the short and long term, are likely to be both material and psychological, and the worry and uncertainty over the future does not invite sound sleep.

Sweden

The threatened closure of a Swedish shipyard in 1988 presented investigators with the unique opportunity of studying the effects of employment instability on sleep patterns. The findings, reported in the *British Medical Journal*[4], were indeed grim. Over 2,500 men were employed at the shipyard at the time of the study. Most of those involved were middle aged, had worked at the shipyard for years and had come to expect ten or more years of a working life to look forward to.

Compared with men of similar ages, who had far better chances of job permanency, the men who lived through a six-year period of protracted negotiations, during which time the future of the shipyard was uncertain, experienced significantly more sleep problems. In addition to this, they were also found to have a greater increase in cholesterol levels and blood pressure. Interestingly, the men with the highest increases in cholesterol also had the most dramatic increases in sleep problems, suggesting that sleep problems intensify in direct relation to the degree of stress present.

Finland

The reality of unemployment in the middle of a national economic slump was again highlighted in the case of Finland in the late 1980s. From the mid-1980s and over a ten-year period, the rate of unemployment in Finland rose from 5 per cent to a staggering 18 per cent across the workforce. Problems of low economic growth, high inflation and unemployment were widespread, with many traditional industries experiencing the worst of the impact. Job prospects, income, and quality and stability of lifestyle were considerably reduced for many of the workers involved. Long-term unemployment was also a real possibility, particularly for middle-aged men, despite their being highly skilled.

Researchers were able to assess the ongoing effects of the economic recession by studying a relatively large representative sample of the population, who had previously submitted health and lifestyle details in a questionnaire distributed prior to this period[5]. Over 1,500 adults took part in this survey, roughly half men and half women. All volunteers were initially approached in the early 1980s during a period of relative economic growth. The questionnaire covered areas of general health concerns: illness, cholesterol levels, drug use (prescribed or otherwise), tobacco and alcohol use, exercise, weight, etc, as well as covering financial and employment details. They were also asked a series of questions about their normal sleeping habits. When did they normally go to bed? Roughly how long did it take them to go to sleep? What time did they normally get up? How frequently were they disturbed during the night, and for what reasons? Did they regularly feel tired or even sleep during the day?

Eight years later, the same volunteers were contacted again. Despite severe economic problems during the intervening years, a comparison of the two questionnaires suggested that for most people sleep patterns were pretty much the same over the eight years.

However, the outcome was not quite so encouraging when particular groups were targeted. More specifically, there was a clear problem of increased insomnia and greater sleep disturbance for those individuals whose daily lives had undergone radical change, due to unemployment or reduced income for example, as a direct result of the prevailing economic situation. These groups were also found to use more sleeping pills, smoke more and report more general fatigue than respondents who remained in fairly stable employment. The most striking problems were found to occur in middle-aged men who had previously been engaged in manual work. Loss of income, in conjunction with low re-employment prospects, was found to be particularly hard-hitting for this group.

UK

A similar effect of job insecurity on disturbed sleep patterns was found for men studied in a British investigation of over 7,500 white-collar workers in the civil service[6]. All participants in this study had clerical roles in government offices in and around London. Extensive medical and survey-type screening was used to assess the effects of job instability during a seven-year period in which their roles within the civil service were under scrutiny for possible transfer to private agencies, with the threat of either redundancy or uncertain future working conditions. In this case, although participants were roughly divided among the sexes, it was only the men who experienced disturbed, usually shortened, sleep.

Why should loss of work affect sleep? The answer to this is perhaps obvious – high levels of anxiety interfere with sleep. Unemployment is generally assumed to be extremely stressful as a result of the insecurity, low income and reduced life prospects, all of which impact on a general sense of well-being. Long-term unemployment can lead to low self-esteem, loss of confidence and a sense of futility. However, work also provides a powerful social zeitgeber by imposing a strict, regular pattern of attendance. This in turn often encourages a certain amount of stability in home life, with fairly regular bedtimes from week to week. One of the effects of losing regular work is that it is up to the individual to find alternative regularity in their lives, if the periods normally allocated to sleep and wake are to remain separate. This is particularly important, given the added problems of sleeping soundly imposed by psychological stress.

Australia

Economic insecurity can have negative consequences for workers in many industries even if it does not necessarily lead to unemployment. Sometimes working conditions change as a result of streamlining or rationalizing within an organization, to the extent that the new demands on employees have a direct effect on their sleep.

In Australia, the late 1980s saw the deregulation of public transport, leading to open competition over routes and prices. In order to compete in an increasingly saturated market, bus companies were forced to embark on a series of cost-cutting exercises. British bus companies experienced a similar change in regulations at about the same time. However, the huge distance between popular destinations in Australia meant that drivers were under increasing pressure to drive on long trips, away from home and sleeping in unfamiliar conditions. The short-term effects of driving while sleepy are potentially catastrophic and rapidly increasing concerns for this area have prompted reviews of driving regulations and legislation (see Chapter 13). In 1991, an Australian group published a survey of male long-distance coach drivers which showed that the build-up over time of working under increasing pressure and the negative effects on general health and family life may have been underestimated[7].

As a group, the drivers were more fatigued than similar men in non-driving occupations, both in the early morning and early evening. Sleep was reduced to an average of less than seven hours per night while working away. Indigestion, irritability and mood complaints were also more prevalent. Of some concern was the reliance on pharmacological stimulants, such as amphetamines, to help with alertness during long stretches of driving, and alcohol to help wind down after a long day. Both of these are known to disturb sleep. Drivers also complained of having to resort to speeding in order to maintain schedules. Overall, levels of work-related stresses were connected directly to sleep disturbance, and perhaps not surprisingly, to accident rates and job dissatisfaction.

Bereavement and divorce

Partners acts as powerful regulators in daily behaviours, perhaps more than we think. Yet for many couples, deciding when to go to bed and when to get up is generally a compromise between both partners' natural rhythms.

Following an abrupt change to this relationship, either through death or divorce, there is often a drawn-out transition period in which sleep patterns adjust to the absence of a partner. In both situations emotional disturbance is likely to be high, and in the short term help with sleep may be necessary. Adaptation can take some time, and may not be complete until such time as the emotional wounds have been dealt with. These concerns are also more likely to be reflected in dream content, which, if particularly disturbing, can leave the person with the impression of having slept badly.

Childbirth

Sleep disturbance is a common complaint during pregnancy, particularly during the first three months and then the final three months before the birth. Expectant mothers are often disturbed in their sleep by the movement of the foetus, heartburn, pressure on the bladder, backache, and more general problems with getting comfortable.

The birth of a baby is also likely to have a dramatic impact on normal sleeping patterns. This may not necessarily be a problem. New parents tend to agree that it is not so much being woken during the night which they find difficult, as the level of unpredictability in the baby's demands. This has been confirmed in studies which show that new mothers can often get just as much sleep over a 24-hour period as before the baby was born, but that it is more likely to be spread out over shorter bursts throughout the day and night, rather than in a single block of seven to eight hours' sleep at night.

During the early weeks, the opportunity to sleep depends largely on the sleep patterns of the baby. Frequent disruptions to short and unpredictable naps can result in severe fatigue, in much the same way as shiftworkers have difficulty operating out of synchrony with the rest of the world. Being woken up unexpectedly is never pleasant, but perhaps even less so if you are faced with this prospect on a nightly basis. Fortunately, for most parents the worst period in terms of sleep disruption is usually the first one to two months and the ability to cope with this is well within their capacity.

One initiative that many parents resort to is to bring the baby into their own bed. This has the advantage, particularly for breastfeeding mothers, of creating fewer disturbances for the parents during the night. It is interesting that many of the earlier concerns for suffocation or 100 per cent demand feeding, popularized by child-care gurus of the 1960s and 1970s, are no longer in vogue. The merits (or otherwise) of bed-sharing with infants are discussed in more detail in Chapter 7.

Natural ageing

Ageing often brings with it complaints of poor sleep, although the reasons for this are unclear. Studies which have looked in detail at the quality of sleep in the elderly tend to confirm these reports, showing among other things a reduction in overall sleep time towards the mid-sixties and beyond. On the whole, sleep tends to be lighter, with less time spent in Stages 3 and 4 sleep. The impact of a change in behaviour following retirement cannot be totally dismissed.

As more and more people can expect to live to old-age, there is now a pressing need to understand the sleep difficulties experienced by the elderly. Of particular concern in the area of natural ageing is how these changes in sleep patterns interact with life events, changes in mobility, health, anxiety and depressive illness.

The menopause

The female menopause has been associated with a decline in sleep quality. Many women find they sleep less soundly during or after the menopause, leading to an overall reduction in sleep – an effect which may go part-way towards explaining changes in mood, especially irritability and fatigue. Hormone replacement therapy (HRT) has been used effectively by many women in dealing with menopausal symptoms, although its effect on sleep problems associated with this syndrome has yet to be established.

Acute stress

Very often, sleep is disturbed following a particularly traumatic event. Distressing imagery and feelings of futility or despair after being involved in or witnessing such an event can make sleep almost impossible, and in extreme cases will warrant the use of sedatives to help with the immediate effects of the experience. Occasionally, problems persist and form part of what is now described as a 'post-traumatic stress syndrome'. Peaceful sleep is only restored when the underlying problems have been dealt with.

This condition can have extremely long-lasting effects. During World War II, a large group of young Frenchmen living in the border town of Alsace between France and Germany were forcibly conscripted into a German military unit, and subsequently fought against the Russian army. Many of them were captured and subjected to extreme hardships in Russian prisoner-of-war camps. Over 40 years later, survivors were identified and contacted by a French team of researchers investigating the long-term effects of severe trauma[8]. Over 1,800 men, most of whom were repatriated by this time and in their mid-sixties, agreed to take part in the investigation. It was found that almost 80 per cent were still experiencing disturbing dreams relating to their experiences in the camp, many including features of their ordeal or direct references to imprisonment, pursuit or the death of fellow prisoners.

While we naturally assume that stress has immediate effects on sleep, long-term stress relating to earlier events, which may have been neglected at the time of their occurrence, is often underestimated and continues to disturb sleep for many years.

Do we need the same amount of sleep every day?

The assumption that most people need to sleep for eight hours a night can have a dispiriting effect on anyone who deviates from this to any extent. This is often due to circumstances beyond their control, and may reflect some underlying personal difficulty. Worries about sleep can only compound the problem, and it is reassurance about being able to cope with reduced sleep that is needed. Being more relaxed with the idea of sleeping less can have a positive effect on quality of sleep.

The health risks associated with sleeping patterns as described earlier in the chapter are intriguing, but it should be noted that these surveys included individuals at both extremes of normal sleeping habits. It may be that factors related to social conditions and lifestyle behaviours (not covered by the investigations), rather than sleep length in itself, were the real source of risk. Changes in sleep patterns can often reflect disturbance in other areas of our life. The recent studies of occupational groups during periods of instability described earlier have shown that sleep disruption is part of a more general physical and behavioural response to a difficult situation.

Ironically, many people get by without eight hours' sleep but do not consider themselves to be at risk. There is even considerable admiration for this type of individual (see Chapter 4). Being able to function effectively on less than eight hours' sleep is a highly prized skill in a busy world, reflecting ambition, dynamism and motivation. In fact, the ability to get by on very little sleep is seen as almost a prerequisite for many professions, with an emphasis on gaining maximum benefit with minimum of time invested in sleep.

Can we sleep too much?

The answer to this question depends on the motivation for sleep at any particular point in time, and can be extremely difficult to assess given the wide range of influences on sleep patterns (see Fig 4). There are two schools of thought in this area. On the one hand, all sleep is seen as important and purposeful: if we are able to do it, then we must need it. This suggests that there is no such thing as oversleeping, but that being able to catch a quick snooze in the afternoon or 'lying in' until past noon on a Sunday is indicative of a genuine physiological need. If you feel yourself regularly veering towards sleep in the afternoon, then this is a behavioural 'cue' to the need to take more sleep at night. What is important, though, is that in this view the environment *facilitates* sleep but does not *cause* it.

Now, on a common-sense level we might like to think that some people are just 'good sleepers', no matter how much sleep they have had – they fall asleep easily, and will probably do so if there is not enough going on around them to keep them awake. For them, activity is the critical factor in remaining awake. We know it works to some extent in extreme circumstances, such as hospital emergency rooms staffed by personnel on round-the-clock shifts. But is the converse also true: is sleep occasionally just a reaction to a lack of activity? What about weekends and holidays – is all this extra sleep necessary, or are we just napping for fun? Choose almost any circumstance where the normal constraints of day-to-day life are removed and we sleep longer.

How much sleep do we need?

The starting point for this discussion is surely: 'Why bother to ask?' Is it not intuitive for us to know whether or not we have had enough sleep, and when to do it? Possibly, but a physiological drive is only part of our decision to sleep. We are now faced with a complex range of powerful influences on activity patterns, which serve to distract us from our need to sleep.

It is also true to say that many people are dissatisfied with their sleep. Sleeping pills and caffeine are used widely throughout the world to customize the habit of sleep to personal circumstance. Sleep disorders are fast gaining recognition as a major source of ill-health.

For a variety of reasons, sleep has been identified as a modern health risk, with good sleep practices (as with diet and exercise) essential for optimum safety and personal efficiency.

Finally, in the absence of the definitive study of sleep patterns, a number of interesting assumptions have emerged. Firstly, stereotypes between cultures and between groups in society remind us of the general intolerance for over-indulgence in sleep. Students and unemployed groups are often assumed to sleep for longer than average, although evidence suggest that these are both stressful conditions that are more likely to result in reduced sleep. Cultural stereotypes are often based on nothing more than the assumption of a strong national work ethic, and population studies have failed to find clear differences in typical sleep patterns between countries.

Another idea, which has proved to be extremely well supported, is the belief that we have undergone an historical change in sleep behaviours over the past 100 years or so. Specifically, we are understood to be sleeping even less than during the Victorian period as a direct result of the significant influence of industrialization, urbanization and the electric light bulb. This is perhaps a little nostalgic, as there is again very little hard evidence to support these claims. It may well be that with a shift from agricultural to industrial activity sleep patterns were simply rearranged, so that waking hours could fit in with the co-ordinated operation of the factory rather than daylight hours.

Are we satisfied with how much sleep we get? Apparently not. A 1991 American Gallup poll estimated that anything up to 40 per cent of the public felt that they were not able to get as much sleep as they needed.

Chapter 6
Getting the timing right

'**A**n hour before midnight is worth two after', or so the saying goes. But is there any truth to it? Well for some people, the answer is definitely yes, but not everybody is ready for sleep quite so early.

This chapter looks at how it can often help to learn to get the timing right before we can expect to go to sleep easily, stay asleep all night and wake up feeling great.

Circadian rhythms

Studies in isolated or artificial-time environments, such as those outlined in earlier chapters, have shown that if you peel away the powerful social and environmental 'time-givers' or zeitgebers, each person has a strong, internally driven 'body clock'. This clock follows a roughly 24½-hour day if allowed to take its own course; in other words, we would choose a day/night period slightly longer than the more natural 24-hour day/night cycle determined by the earth's rotation around the sun. We describe the influence of this internal clock as following a 'circadian' pattern.

Throughout a complete daily cycle we swing between highs and lows of alertness and sleepiness. This happens no matter how much sleep we have had, or how much we've missed. For example, even after a night without sleep, by mid-morning the next day the pressure for sleep is starting to ease and most people will be feeling reasonably fine by this point. Sleepiness is typically at its most extreme in the middle of the night, with a second low spot in the mid-afternoon. We can think of these as 'troughs' in the daily alertness cycle. These contrast with 'peaks' in alertness at around mid-morning and early evening.

As well as fluctuations in the urge to sleep throughout the 24-hour period, this rhythm is also evident in the ability actually to fall asleep and sleep soundly. That is why it is often difficult to sleep through the morning despite being up all night – a problem many shiftworkers have to deal with.

Due to the regularity and predictability of this internal daily rhythm, there are times when we feel awake because it is the right 'time' to be awake and not simply because we are refreshed from sleep. So after working straight through a night shift, it is normal to begin to pick up again by morning and feel more 'awake' and refreshed, even without the benefit of sleep. Most of us are 'day' creatures – all our body functions favour being at our best during this time and, conversely, work towards providing the optimal conditions for getting the most out of an inactive period at night.

As well as a regular sleepiness drive, there are a number of other biological functions which follow a strong daily pattern. These include changes in body temperature and the release of adrenalin, melatonin and human growth hormone. Basic psychological functions such as memory and deductive reasoning skills also fluctuate across a 24-hour period; at night, when sleepiness is at its greatest, even simple 'brain teasers' may take extra effort or time to complete.

As the circadian rhythm of body temperature has been shown to be extremely important in relation to the sleepiness rhythm, monitoring hour-by-hour fluctuations in temperature has helped to shed light on why some sleep periods are more satisfying than others. Given the opportunity, most people prefer to sleep on a schedule of late evening to early morning. This usually coincides with a gradual decrease in body temperature towards bedtime and a steady rise again in early morning. When in synchrony like this, the relationship between sleep and temperature can help to predict ease of sleeping and satisfaction. If we try to sleep at any other point on the temperature cycle – for example, as it rises further through mid-morning – then this interferes with the ability to fall asleep, and makes for short, light and easily disturbed sleep, if any at all.

Owls and larks

'Early to bed, early to rise, makes a man, healthy, and wise'. Well, that might be stretching it a bit too far, but it does give some idea of the way in which societies, old and new, have favoured people who function at their best first thing in the morning.

Some people prefer to be up bright and early in the morning, but are reluctant to stay up late at night without good reason. Others just can't seem to say goodbye to the day, and will stay up way past midnight despite an inevitable struggle to get out of bed the next morning. Are these differences in sleep patterns a question of habit, personal preference, personality or lifestyle? Is it all a matter of training and self-discipline?

The evidence suggests that these differences are in fact genuine and reflect extremes in the body's own circadian rhythms in relation to the earth's day/night cycles. People who function best in the morning (we can describe these as 'larks') actually start to feel sleepier earlier on in the night, and not just because they have been up for longer. This is more obvious when it is necessary to cut back on sleep. Larks find it easier to get up an hour earlier than normal if necessary, and are less keen to stay up later than normal. The converse is true for night 'owls', who have extreme difficulty when faced with an early start in the morning, but are much happier with extending the day if necessary. Owls would struggle to sleep if they went to bed that bit earlier in the evening, while larks would not. The typical bedtimes, sleepiness and alertness zones for these two extremes are illustrated in Fig 5.

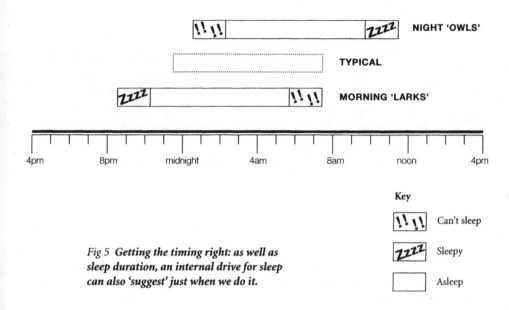

Fig 5 **Getting the timing right: as well as sleep duration, an internal drive for sleep can also 'suggest' just when we do it.**

The sleepiness/alertness rhythm tends to be more inflexible for larks, who cannot lie in the next day as well as owls can – even after a late night. If owls have a late night, they just make up for it by staying in bed that bit longer in the morning. So perhaps we should have more sympathy for 'night owls' who really cannot cope with getting up in the morning, and for 'larks' who always seem to be desperate for sleep just when the party's starting.

Of course, only a small proportion of the population are at these two extremes; most people are aware of preferring one end of the day to the other, but within limits are usually quite flexible – for example, most people who live together go to bed at around the same time. There is also a serious side to this issue, though, as more and more people are being asked to sleep outside their normal sleep rhythm, usually to accommodate work arrangements. Some people find it easier to cope with work throughout the 24-hour cycle and tolerate shiftwork much better than others. As you might expect, night owls tend to have an advantage over larks when it comes to working at night, and may find this rescheduling of sleep and work less of a problem. The problem lies, not so much with staying awake during the night – this can be dealt with by staying active – but in trying to sleep during the day. It seems that the lark may be less flexible than the owl and cannot simply fall asleep at the drop of a hat.

As well as sleeping, owls and larks also regulate their daily behaviours around different timings for eating, work, leisure and social activities. However, these lark and owl behaviour patterns are not necessarily fixed for life, but can change subject to age, lifestyle and one's frame of mind (eg depressive illness).

Age factors

It has been pointed out that owl and lark tendencies are also reflected in well known behavioural patterns which coincide with distinct periods in life, particular around early adolescent and middle to old age. Parents fight a losing battle to get their teenager to go to bed earlier so that they can at least get up in the morning, while the elderly often complain about waking up too early and not being able to get back to sleep.

With the transition to these ages, although there is a subtle shift in sleep patterns towards these arrangements, it is often difficult to isolate the effects of a change in internal drives from the pressing social factors that also emerge at these times. For teenagers, these changes in sleep patterns towards more 'owl-like' behaviours may be triggered by a move away from parental control towards increased autonomy, and more adult, peer-defined bedtimes. Again, the combined effects of changes in physiological and social factors on sleep patterns are also apparent for the elderly. With increasing age comes a weakening of circadian rhythms, possibly as a breakdown in synchrony between the basic functions governing sleep, and often in combination with additional physical discomfort due to spending long periods in the same position (weakened bladder, poor circulation), or problems of poor health and chronic pain. Typical age-related sleep complaints include more awakenings during the night, difficulty in getting to sleep, sleepiness and unscheduled napping during the day, and an increased tendency towards 'lark-type' sleep patterns (which is often only really a problem in relation to early-morning awakenings). The elderly are also faced with a weakening of social zeitgebers, as they move beyond a working life and face the challenge of replacing these influences with equally powerful routines or regulators.

As we get older, it is thought that circadian rhythms change in two ways – in their relationship with other rhythms, and in strength – both of which can have some knock-on effect on the quality and experience of sleep. It has been suggested that the peaks and troughs of the day's sleepiness rhythm are 'ironed-out' with increasing age, so that the extremes of being very tired or very alert are no longer felt; consequently, it is harder to get to sleep at night, actual sleep is lighter (there is very little Stage 3 and 4 sleep compared with young adults), it is more easily disturbed, and it doesn't last as long. This disruption in sleep tends to occur earlier in women than in men, with early signs in the forties and fifties, although hormonal changes coinciding with this age and/or differences in a willingness to report or complain about sleep may be partially responsible for the recording of such differences.

Shiftwork

Shiftworkers often have to deal with extreme difficulties brought about by fighting against their natural rhythms, in order to stay awake at a time that is convenient and necessary for them to work. The difficulties in achieving this centre around problems of attempting to sleep and stay awake during the wrong times of the peaks and troughs of the circadian alertness rhythm. Although some adaptation is possible, additional problems emerge with rotating shifts (ie changing from morning to afternoon to night shifts), which present the worker with a new sleep/wake/work schedule at regular intervals, sometimes weeks or even only days apart. Even permanent night-shift workers are in a constant state of flux because of the many daytime distractions which interfere with their ability to get a good 'day's' sleep, and the pressure to follow a more 'normal' pattern of night-sleeping on days off.

Apart from sleepiness and alertness, the shiftworker might also experience a range of social and physiological difficulties. Sleeping during the day can interfere with appetite and normal eating habits, as the night worker may not feel like a large meal shortly after waking up in the late afternoon. The body normally expects to digest food during the day: if we follow good eating habits, then the body signals the behavioural cue for food (hunger pangs), at roughly the same time each day and produces digestive juices in anticipation of a meal. This can cause difficulties, as eating habits necessarily follow from other behaviours, including sleeping and work patterns. In particular, the body is not normally prepared for eating at night, during which time heavy meals can take longer to digest and lead to the discomfort of indigestion. A heavy, high-fat meal can also increase the effects of sleepiness during the night. Although night-shift workers are often advised to eat light snacks of low-fat, non-stodgy foods if they cannot avoid eating altogether on a night shift, there may well be a strong social pressure during the shift to do other-wise – as if this were a normal work period with a long break half-way to accommodate 'lunch'.

To help with the transition between shifts, particularly on to a series of night shifts, workers are often advised to ease the circadian system into a more gentle rather than abrupt transition. In preparation for a series of night shifts, workers might try going to bed later and later, with a short daytime sleep before the first night shift to help them get through the night. On sub-sequent days, although it is important to get as much sleep as possible, this can often be difficult to achieve because of the conflicting messages between the body's need to sleep (due to being awake all night), a circadian drive for alertness (as the mid-morning 'peak' is approached), social pressure to stay awake (family, friends, hobbies), and environmental sleep inhibitors (noise, sunlight, temperature). The net result of this competition between sleep factors is that the shiftworker can often have a very hard time getting sufficient sleep during the day to cope with being awake, and working, all night.

Researchers have been working with a variety of measures to improve conditions for the shiftworker. For example, it is known that avoiding bright sunlight during the early morning, before expecting to go to sleep, can help with sleeping during the day. Conversely, the night-shift worker is advised to go out into the sunshine during the early evening. The precise reasons for the success of using bright light to manage sleepiness drives are as yet unclear, although the role of light as a powerful natural zeitgeber in determining sleep/wake patterns has been known for some time. The introduction of artificial bright light, timed to coincide with a critical phase of the circadian sleepiness rhythm, has been found to be effective for a wide range of sleep timing problems, some of which are relatively modern concerns (such as shiftwork or jet lag) while others are related to features of the natural environment (seasonal affective disorder – the winter blues).

Shiftworkers are also advised to avoid strong caffeinated drinks towards the end of the night shift, or alcohol before going to sleep during the day or starting a night shift. Alcohol is not an effective sleep aid, because it disrupts the restorative quality of sleep. In addition to this, alcohol also impairs reactions and leads to drowsiness – factors that can exacerbate the difficulties experienced in staying awake throughout the night.

Circadian rhythm disorders

Occasionally, the daily internal rhythms governing a drive to sleep and wake are either so far removed from the 24-hour pattern of normal activity or set for such an odd time that the individual can find themselves in need of help. Serious problems with circadian rhythms make life unbearable, due to the resulting competition between following a preferred pattern of daily activity and that governed by the body. One example of such a condition is known as Delayed Sleep Phase Syndrome (DSPS), in which the daily rhythm is set much later than usual to produce extreme night owls. Often, sufferers of DSPS also find themselves running on a slightly longer day (25 hours, for example), with the result that they feel the need to go to bed later and later each night and wake up later each morning.

It can often be difficult to recognize this as a problem: as with long and short sleepers, many people tend to see sleep patterns as a matter of choice. It may therefore be assumed that the 'night owl' who stays up all night partying has only themselves to blame for being late to work in the morning. This may be true in many cases, but from time to time the problems are of a more genuine physiological nature involving the timing of the circadian system.

This syndrome is perhaps more common than is realized and it has only recently come to the attention of medical practitioners, possibly due to the introduction of more effective treatments in this area. It is often hidden by lifestyles lacking in social zeitgebers, where such unusual sleep patterns would be relatively easier to tolerate – for example, during college years or for self-employed professions where the individual has more freedom to dictate their own work hours. Difficulties may only emerge when that person is forced to adapt their sleep hours to a more conventional, regular pattern, such as that necessitated by a new job requiring traditional 'office hours'.

DSPS is not the same as going to bed late out of choice – people who do that are able to make a big effort and go to bed earlier and actually sleep earlier if and when circumstances change, whereas going to bed early is often ineffective for the DSPS sufferer, as it can take hours for them to go to sleep and getting up in the morning is rarely improved by this strategy. There are two reasons for this: firstly, there is the acute fatigue of a relatively short night's sleep, and secondly, because the 'body clock' is set to a later timing, the body is simply not ready to be awake at that time in the day. As a result, there is often a constant battle to stay away during the day, with additional problems in daily life which can include difficulties with concentration or mood, and effects on performance at school, work and social activities.

The problem of rescheduling the timing of the circadian rhythm of sleepiness in these cases can be dealt with in a number of ways. With chronotherapy, for example, the DSPS sufferer is advised to go to bed later each night (usually by two to three hours), sleep or stay in bed for eight hours, and then get up. Over a matter of days, this shifts bedtimes across the whole day. Eventually (after about a week) bedtimes move closer to the desired time and will hopefully be maintained from then on, although regular resetting in this way may be necessary. Extending the day with this method is found to be easier than attempting to impose an abrupt change, as the individual is at least sleepy when they go to bed, although in the short term there is the considerable inconvenience of sleeping at unusual times. This can often further isolate the DSPS sufferer, who must reorganize their activity schedule during the course of the treatment.

In extreme cases, when the circadian 'day' length follows a cycle much longer than the normal 24-hour period (ie an extra one to two hours is tagged on the end of each 'natural' day and sleep/wake patterns gradually shift around the 24-hour day), the DSPS sufferer is further out of synchrony with the rest of their immediate social group and may need to find the ongoing treatment to which they are best suited in order to deal with this situation.

Bright light treatment (usually timed in the middle of the night) has also been found to be an effective intervention for some people and can help to prepare the body for an earlier awakening, although waking to administer the treatment is in itself extremely difficult for the DSPS sufferer. This approach has also been used for Advanced Sleep Phase Syndrome (ASPS), another circadian-related problem, in which the sufferer finds themselves exhausted and in need of sleep by early evening, but unable to sleep beyond early morning. This condition, although more unusual than DSPS, has been treated effectively by using bright light to stay awake that bit longer in the evening, thereby rescheduling the sleepiness rhythm to a later time.

Bright light treatment, now commercially available, has the advantage of being drug-free, although self-discipline is required in order to administer treatment at the right time and for sufficient duration for it to be effective.

Is there a 'wrong' side of the bed?

The relationship between sleep and mood is a complex and intriguing one. We often talk about 'getting out of the wrong side of the bed' in order to describe bad moods in the morning which appear to have no obvious cause, and follow even after a normal night of sleep. Interestingly, with depressed in-patients considerable effort has been put into developing treatments aimed at manipulating the timing and duration of sleep at night with a view to improving mood, at least in the short term. In these cases, researchers have found quite a striking effect of sleep deprivation on mood, suggesting that there is indeed a relationship between how we feel in the morning and the process of sleep. However, as common sense suggests, it is not simply a question of getting enough sleep, as bad tempers and depressed moods often show themselves when people sleep for their normal seven or eight hours at night, or perhaps even longer.

It has been suggested that the secret to this lies in getting the timing right, and that we wake up feeling our best when this moment coincides with other rhythms in the body which help to prepare us for the demands of the day. This is, perhaps, particularly the case for body temperature, which shows a gradual rise as the body prepares for wake during the later part of the night. It seems that we feel at our best if we time our waking-up to coincide with the general warming of the body. At any other time we are less than comfortable, and this is especially so if we try to wake up during the dip in body temperature. So, better quality sleep and how we feel as we wake up is often related to the timing of waking rather than the length of sleep. For example, if we prefer to ignore the first cue to wake up at the weekends and decide to sleep on, then two hours further down the line we can actually wake up feeling worse than before: thick-headed, sleepy, and not in the best of moods.

Chapter 7
Propaganda for kids?

Adequate sleep, along with good nutrition and a favourable environmental and social conditions, is generally considered to be an essential staple of the developmental 'diet' in modern western societies. It is, therefore, the responsibility of the parents to provide the necessary conditions throughout childhood for regular, undisturbed sleep. The idea that sleep 'training' is an essential part of the socialization process is fundamental to most childcare practices. Being able to sleep well is a 'skill' considered to be as important an indication of normal development in other key areas of achievement, such as toilet training and weaning on to solid foods. At the back of most parents' minds is the vague idea that sleep is essential for normal growth, and the fact that children's sleep is deeper and usually longer than that of most adults would seem to support this idea. However, exactly how much sleep children need across the various stages of their development is open to question.

Child-care practices are modified with almost every new generation of parents. Over the years, it is clear that the ideas about what is good for a child are largely dependent on current social and economic contexts. The role of the mother, in particular, will depend to a great extent on the attitude of the labour market towards women at the time. Thus, new or sometimes rehashed ideas about feeding and sleeping arrangements are quickly passed on through ante-natal care, midwives and parental support groups. Mothers and daughters within the same family can be faced with conflicting 'official' advice on key issues of child-care over a relatively short span of time. The critical question, as with many areas of child development, is how far social conditions, including parental behaviours, influence the emergence of biological properties, such as the capacity to maintain sleep over a long period. Do we integrate the two factors effectively and sensibly in order to produce optimum conditions for children's sleep?

Concerns for children's sleep and welfare extend way beyond the years of infancy. For school-aged children, the link between educational achievement and sleep at night has always been a major issue. At the moment, the worry is that children's bedrooms are so well equipped with televisions, videos and computer games that children remain awake way beyond ideal bedtimes. As a consequence of these distractions, it is argued that repeated late nights affect mood and performance in the classroom, as the child is either unable or unwilling to pay attention for long periods simply because they are feeling so sleepy.

If left to their own devices, most children would prefer not to go to bed at the time set by parents. But unlike adults, children tend to respond differently to being short of sleep. Very young children, for instance, are often invigorated by staying up late and will race around full of energy as if sleep is the last thing they need. On top of this, it is exceedingly difficult to know what is normal for every particular child because of the wide range of individual needs, even at an early age. Unfortunately it is all too easy for parents to feel inadequate or out of control when things go wrong.

This chapter looks at some of the specific current issues concerning children's sleep and parenting styles and explores the particular concerns about sleep at each developmental stage.

Babies

The first few weeks

We are told that following birth most babies can be expected to sleep for between 15 and 16 hours a day. This is highly unpredictable and never to be guaranteed, as there is an enormous amount of variation from one baby to the other, even between babies in the same family. Some babies seem to do nothing but sleep and feed for the first few months of their life; these are often described as 'contented' babies by their parents. At the other extreme, there are babies who sleep very little, particularly during the day, when they are easily distracted by noise and activity. Both extremes are normal and have their advantages. Many parents get an inkling of their baby's sleep preferences during the first few days and nights.

After just a couple of weeks, there is often a definite shift towards sleeping more at night and less during the day. An obvious explanation for this is that the house tends to be quieter at this time, with less movement both inside and out. Babies, although still only sleeping for three to four hours at a stretch, tend to sleep more during the early hours of the night.

This is perhaps the first opportunity for parents to assert their own preferences. What constitutes a 'reasonable' bedtime for some parents may seem outrageous to others, and depends largely on how determined parents are to have the evening to themselves. Some babies will be quite happy to go to bed at 7pm or 8pm, although the trade-off for the parents is likely to be an early start in the morning. On the other hand, for the sake of a peaceful undisturbed night, a baby who is quite happy to stay awake without being demanding or disruptive will often be allowed to do so until the parents are ready for bed themselves. There are obviously no right or wrong answers here, and it is up to the individual parents to try to establish a routine with which they feel comfortable. Unfortunately, this compromise between parents and baby is not always easy to achieve to everyone's satisfaction.

Problems can emerge at any stage, even when babies have previously shown a reliable and regular pattern. This is particularly frustrating for parents whose baby insists on reverting to night-waking after spending the previous two to three months sleeping through the night. This can sometimes be traced to an initial disruption, such as a brief illness, teething problems or an abrupt change in the immediate environment, although it soon develops into a sleeping 'issue' between parents and baby beyond the original problem. In these cases, the preferred pattern needs to be re-established and the baby's innate drive for sleep brought into step with positive social influences. This becomes easier as the baby matures physically, and many parents regard their baby's sleep pattern at six to nine months as fairly stable and well established.

Transitions in other areas of development, particularly language and mobility, often coincide with an adjustment in sleep patterns. The ability to cope with longer periods of fasting between feeds also tends to coincide with more consolidated periods of sleep rather than short but frequent naps. The expectation, certainly in many western societies, is that within the first three months a baby should be sleeping straight through the night, with one or two short, supplementary naps during the day.

Why do babies cry so much?

It is often thought that problems arise because of parents' expectations of the baby's sleep patterns during the first year. Crying, especially over long periods during the day or night, can be extremely frustrating for the parent in charge, while understanding the reasons for crying is often a hit-and-miss process. After the obvious possibilities such as feeding, winding, changing and inspecting for injury have been dealt with, it is natural to assume that a crying baby is in need of sleep. This is an even more likely possibility if crying occurs at regular times during the day. Yet parents often claim that some babies simply cry more than others, and that differences crop up even within the same family when many factors remain equal.

Between 1978 and 1980 over 200 pregnant women from the central Manchester area in England were invited to take part in a study looking into infant crying patterns throughout the first year of life[1]. The study was to begin following the delivery of their baby. The women were then asked to provide a 'snapshot' of their baby's behaviour across a 24-hour period, taking detailed records of all periods of crying, sleeping, feeding, bathing, going out on trips and peaceful waketime. This was repeated on selected days at regular intervals throughout the year. The main focus of the study was to try to find out if there were any obvious differences in home or family circumstances that led some babies to cry more than others throughout this potentially stressful period. The main findings confirmed, reassuringly, a gradual decline in the amount of time babies spent crying from birth to their first birthday. There was also, as many parents won't need telling, a marked difference in the extent of crying from one baby to another. No obvious explanation could be found for this in terms of birth order, social factors, financial stability, housing or parental relationships. On average, at six weeks old mothers reported between four and five fairly sustained crying episodes throughout the 24-hour period. Most of this occurred during the night. By one year old, this was reduced to less than two crying episodes. What was interesting, however, was that the babies who cried more than usual at six weeks continued to do so throughout the rest of the year.

There are a number of possible explanations for this, the most obvious being to do with temperament and parental response. By identifying a baby as particularly demanding early on, this may lead parents and care-givers to modify their way of handling the baby to reinforce this behaviour. However, this is an extremely difficult assumption to make as the range of physiological, social or environmental factors that influence parent/infant interactions is huge.

Breastfeeding emerged in a positive light, with those babies who were breastfed throughout the trial being more likely to cry less than formula-fed babies. Again, the reasons for this are unclear: both interactional differences between baby and mother and qualitative differences in the type of feed offer possible explanations.

Many parents report, anecdotally, that second and third babies settle more quickly into a night-time routine. It may be assumed that experienced parents are less likely to reinforce crying for no good reason by not 'rewarding' children with their presence at the first cry or handling them until they fall back to sleep. Yet birth order was not found to be a determining factor in this study.

In the early months, many parents find that their babies become especially demanding during the later afternoon, and will fuss and cry as if tired but refuse to sleep or feed. This is sometimes described as a 'six o'clock colic' and is a phase quite common in babies of two to four months old. There is no difference between bottle-fed or breastfed babies in reports of this disturbance. It may be that at around this time the baby is sensitive to the transition between day and night, ie a change in the light, activity in the home, meals being prepared, perhaps anxiety in the care-giver. Fortunately, this phase is over relatively quickly for most babies.

Is routine important?

There has never been a shortage of 'expert' advice on how to deal with difficult baby issues. Most of these reinforce the belief in establishing regularity and routine in daily activities if the baby is to 'learn' that the night-time is for sleep and nothing else. In the 1960s and 1970s in particular, great emphasis was placed on parenting skills if the baby was to be integrated successfully into the family. Parents were warned not to allow themselves to be at the 'beck and call' of the baby's every whim. They were to be suspicious of the motivations of a well fed, dry and comfortable baby who persisted in waking through the night beyond six months of age. Over-dependence on the physical presence of parents during the night, encouraged by excessive rocking, singing and cradling, particularly in the middle of the night, was considered to be counterproductive in the long run. Instead, it was thought that babies should be encouraged to be more self-sufficient from an early age. They should be allowed to spend time on their own and become independent to the point where they would sleep comfortably in a room of their own, and even be able to soothe themselves back off to sleep if necessary.

Attempts to encourage babies to sleep through the night by appeasement can often backfire. Heavy feeds before putting the baby down are likely to lead to more soiling and wetter babies by the middle of the night, who will then wake and demand changing. The 'quick' feed in the night, to soothe them and help them get back off to sleep can soon establish a routine.

Often when things appear to be going well, a baby will relapse and re-introduce night-wakings, with demands for drinks or cuddles. This is quite a normal turn of events even for babies who are quite a bit older, perhaps into their second year, and can quickly develop into a battle of wills in which both parties are determined not to give in. It also seems that there is quite a fragile balance between sleep habits and sleep need, with many changes throughout this time.

When a baby starts to crawl, take an interest in the outside world and develop a wider social circle, this may have noticeable effects on sleep. Without language, it is difficult to establish with any certainty when children first begin to dream as we understand it. Freud suggested that the very first dreams are basic, factual extensions of the waking experience and only begin to develop their adult-like complexity with emotional and psychological maturation. Bad dreams, though, are apparent quite early on and may be a source of disturbed sleep which parents should look out for, even though the child struggles to articulate their anxieties. Anxiety over separation from the mother in particular is often cited as the source of early dream-related disturbances.

Where should babies sleep?

As babies show an awareness of their surroundings from a very early age, it may be kinder to encourage them to fall asleep in the same place they are going to find themselves in if they wake up during the night. That way, they are less likely to be alarmed or surprised to wake in a strange room, all alone in the dark. Babies who are cuddled or rocked to sleep will eventually need to be transferred to a cold bed and many, not surprisingly, object to this sudden change in environment by waking shortly afterwards. The problem with this approach to bedtime is that the baby is never offered the opportunity to feel comfortable and safe in their own bed, and will object to finding themselves abandoned by their parents after being so lovingly cradled to sleep. In these situations, negative associations with the bedtime routine quickly develop for both the baby and parents.

Is bed-sharing a good idea?

Until recently, parents were advised that under no circumstances should babies be allowed to sleep in the parental bed. This was to be one of the 'golden rules' of western child-care practice. Apart from the presumed risk of suffocation, the idea of the mother being in constant attendance for the baby was untenable. Even as a coping strategy for extremely difficult babies, this was not generally considered to be a realistic option, and resorting to this measure through desperation reflected badly on parenting skills.

However, lately there has been a considerable shift in thinking in this area, so that many western parents now adopt co-sleeping, or bed-sharing with their very young babies as a preferred arrangement, particularly in the first few weeks or months. Concerns about suffocation are less of an issue, unless there are other factors involved, such as alcohol, smoking or over-crowding. This has perhaps coincided with a more general change in attitudes towards baby-care, in which the presumed underlying power struggles between baby and parent are less of a concern, to be replaced by a more infant-centred approach. For some parents, bed-sharing, as with extended breastfeeding on demand, is not seen as a last resort but as a normal and cherished part of bringing up a family. Bed-sharing has obvious benefits in reducing family stress, as parents are more relaxed and feel more assured of getting a better night's sleep. So many parents are now willing to entertain the idea of bed-sharing that bed manufacturers have been quick to respond with the production of a 'family-size' bed.

But do babies and parents actually sleep better all in the same bed? Very little research has been conducted in this area. At the time of deciding to take the baby into their own bed, parents may think that nothing could possibly be worse than their current situation, while at the back of their minds they may be wondering whether this is a decision they will later regret.

Of the few studies which have looked at quality of sleep, it has been shown that mothers and babies do actually sleep 'lighter' when they sleep together. This is not necessarily a bad thing, though, as there may be benefits in terms of reassurance and reduced anxiety for the mother from sleeping with 'one eye open', even though this interferes with overall quality of sleep. The mother is comforted by having the baby close by, with many claiming to be sensitive to changes in their baby's position, temperature, breathing, etc even while they are both asleep. The mother and baby also usually sleep face to face and in close proximity for most of the night, thus allowing the mother to 'monitor' the sleeping baby.

Babies who are breastfed and allowed to sleep with their mothers tend to feed more often throughout the night, and for shorter periods, although this causes only minimal disruption to the mother's sleep as she is not required to get up to attend to the baby. Researchers point out that this arrangement offers a more naturalistic feeding pattern during the night. Also, the baby is comforted almost immediately, rather than having to scream loud enough to be heard from their own room, causing less distress to older children and partners.

It is clear from recent favourable studies that there has been a distinct shift in opinion over the last 20 years or so. Being physically close to an infant throughout the first one to two years is no longer considered to be such a threat to personal space and independence, as is already the case for many cultures where co-sleeping has always been a way of life. It is, after all, only in the last 150–200 years that western babies have been separated at a very early age from their mothers during sleep.

Although more and more families are taking this route, obviously not all parents are willing to entertain the idea of bed-sharing because of the intrusion into their own free time and space. The popularity and success of bed-sharing goes some way towards undermining conventional views on baby sleep, in which it has long been assumed that a baby can only achieve restful, undisturbed sleep when it is lying still in a quiet, darkened room. Yet the newborn baby is surely familiar with noise, both inside and outside the mother's body, close physical contact and movement, and may find these conditions reassuring – conditions which are much closer to a bed-sharing arrangement than the peace, quiet and isolation of a nursery.

In many areas of the world, co-sleeping with a young baby can have genuine advantages by creating a bond between mother and child, providing physical protection in potentially hostile environments and enabling a naturalistic pattern of feeding. However, despite renewed interest in bed-sharing, most American mothers do not sleep with their newborn babies. Instead, the mother usually sleeps near to her baby during the first one to two weeks, but then prefers to move the baby out into a separate room. The reasons for this are complicated, reflecting a concern that both mother and baby are in need of early separation if the baby is to develop a sense of independence, and the mother is to regain hers. Instead, more emphasis is placed on bedtime routines, such as reading, cuddling and singing, as an alternative to sleeping together. It is also very common for the child to be offered a maternal replacement, usually a soft toy or soother, which they can become highly dependent on as a sleeping partner and an object of love. This idea of displacing affection on to a substitute focus epitomizes the western dilemma:

does the baby need somebody or something to share love and closeness during the night, and if so, how much is enough?

Growing up

When is it time to give up the afternoon nap?

It may be surprising to know that in China it is fairly common for half an hour of the school timetable to be set aside in the early afternoon for students to have a short sleep, right up to high-school level[2]

This is not the case in many western countries, where the value of an afternoon nap and its effect on sleep at night becomes a real issue when a child reaches about four to five years of age. By five years it is generally expected that most children will no longer rely on a daily afternoon nap. This also coincides with starting school, and many educational systems are reluctant to allow children to sleep during the day beyond this age.

As children become gradually 'weaned' from their nap, this can often be a time of stress for the parent. The impression is that there is a distinct 'window' of opportunity during the day for the nap which, if missed, can have repercussions for behaviour during the early evening. By four or o'clock in the afternoon a child who has for some reason decided to go without a nap that day may become unbearably cranky. Allowing the child to sleep at this point, although tempting, will almost definitely cause problems later.

The propensity to nap during the afternoon stays with most of us throughout adulthood, although the social norm may discourage us from giving in to it. In young children, though, the fact that many will actually sleep in the afternoon if given the opportunity to do so suggests that getting a good night's sleep is more important than ever.

Are there problems with school work after a late night?

As children get older, parents are regularly and predictably faced with the all too familiar challenge: 'Why do I have to go to bed?' Children grumble and moan their way through the same old protests night after night: 'I'm not tired.' 'My friends always stay up later.' 'I promise to get up in the morning.' 'How long is she staying up for?' 'That's not fair!'

At around this time parents often make one crucial mistake – to hint that bedtimes might be negotiable! From this point on there is no turning back and the scene is set for a nightly struggle. In this way, we customarily 'train' children to think that bedtime routines are open-ended – stories, drinks, chatting and cuddles – and complain when we lose control. Putting a child to bed might be a valuable opportunity for 'quality' interaction between parent and child, but it can so often backfire. Children not only have to be ready for sleep, but they should also be willing. A dysfunctional bedtime routine can often interfere with this willingness.

Eventually, for some children, all the whining pays off, and they manage to persuade their parents that it is 'cool' for them to follow their own 'rhythm' and decide for themselves when they are ready for bed. It's a nice idea, but unfortunately children do not have a normal 'adult' reaction to tiredness. Tiredness and fatigue can even seem to generate activity in young children.

Nowadays, although we accept the need for children to get a good night's sleep if they are to cope intellectually and socially with the challenges of the school day, in practice this is not always easy to achieve. Historically, sleep in children has been an educational issue from around the turn of this century. The first real drive towards understanding how much sleep children need coincided with a more general interest in educational aptitude, an issue which was to take on more and more importance with the advent of education for all in many countries. This was fuelled to a great extent by developments in child psychology and the introduction of standardized intelligence testing.

A large number of studies took place in different countries throughout the world over a 20-year period, with two American researchers, Lewis Terman and Adeline Hocking, being particularly influential in this area. At the time, Terman was also the driving force behind the development of what was to become one of the most widely used techniques for measuring intelligence: the Stanford-Binet intelligence test. This technique allowed large numbers of children to be measured and compared along a scale of intellectual ability. In their pioneering studies of American schoolchildren which took place from around 1910 onwards, Terman and Hocking looked specifically at maturational changes in sleep patterns and how this was related to intellectual development[3].

Everyday factors, such as distractions from siblings, shared bedrooms, heat, noise and social pressure, were all taken into account in trying to establish why it was that children slept for different lengths of time at night. (Distraction from the activities of other family members, particularly siblings, has been thought to present difficulties in allowing children to follow individual preferences for sleep, particularly if the same bedroom is being shared by children of very different ages. The evidence suggests that, particularly for younger siblings, bedtimes get later and later depending on the number of children in the family.) Similar studies were already underway, or planned, in European countries, where the same concerns were being voiced. From the tone of these reports, it is clear that around this time many researchers were already worried about the consequences of children not getting enough sleep.

The natural assumption has always been that sleep is beneficial in terms of intellectual development in children and so researchers, quite reasonably, expected to find some relationship between sleep length and school achievement. Terman and Hocking followed this line of argument by comparing sleep length with (1) educational success, (2) personality traits and (3) social conditions. Over 2,500 children and young adults were studied, either directly or with the help of parents and teachers, to establish their normal patterns of sleep. To the apparent surprise of both authors, no link was found between how much sleep the children had at night and their level of educational attainment across the range of school subjects, or with overt personality traits, such as nervousness or timidity, or conditions at home.

We have nevertheless been reluctant to give up on the idea that children need a good night's sleep, and that those who are unable to get this, for whatever reason, will be disadvantaged in daily life, particularly at school. It may simply be that the children involved in this study were genuinely not at risk. What did emerge from this investigation, though, was a suspicion that children's sleep varied from country to country. For that reason, Terman and Hocking included in their report an extensive account of contemporary investigations of children's sleep, showing considerable discrepancies between studies. Different techniques for gathering information go some way towards explaining these discrepancies, although underlying cultural differences in beliefs about children's sleep patterns could not be ruled out.

German, Danish and English studies all found that six-year-olds tended to sleep for around 10–11 hours per night, but disagreed on the rate at which children reduced their sleep as they got older, with some following more 'adult' patterns at a relatively early age. For example, English girls seemed to be sleeping as little as seven-and-a-half hours per night by the age of 13. This was a concern for researchers working on the study, who estimated that at 13 years old children needed much closer to 11 hours sleep per night. Often it was the case that home backgrounds or institutional restrictions played a part in guiding habitual sleep lengths, despite there being very little hard evidence concerning the physiological requirements for sleep across the development span. This led to some particularly harsh schedules. For instance, a survey of British boarding schools around this time revealed that pupils as young as 10 years old were restricted to as little as eight or nine hours' sleep per night.

In contrast, the American children studied by Terman and Hocking were found to sleep quite a bit longer (about an hour and a half on average) than European children, a fact which puzzled the investigators and led to speculation concerning the temperate Californian climate. It was suggested that this allowed the American children to lead a more active, outdoor lifestyle, with subsequent benefits for sleep. Also, Californian schools started an hour later than many European schools, allowing children more time in bed in the morning. The possibility that social class was a factor in determining sleep length for children was considered, with the European studies being drawn from less affluent, more industrialized sectors. This factor has more recently been found to be an important issue, with substantive evidence of the effects of lifestyles, poverty and large families on determining children's sleep. To assess whether children are in fact getting enough sleep, we need to consider what it is they are doing to make them stay up so late.

Distractions from sleep – why argue?

Today, more and more children expect to have a television, videos and computer games in their bedrooms, which might keep them a bit quieter but they are probably not asleep. Not surprisingly, the television is often blamed for distracting children from their homework or keeping them up beyond a reasonable bedtime. However, there is not an awful lot of evidence for this. In one of the most substantial recent studies in this area, researchers failed to endorse this view, and found that hours spent in front of a television did not seem to have a negative effect on sleep duration for young children[4]. Again, the evidence is sparse, and it often fails to represent a broad range of social conditions.

That children might be distracted from sleep by circumstantial factors is by no means a recent concern. In the early 1930s, researchers Renshaw, Marquis and Miller from the Universities of Yale and Ohio were faced with similar worries, not with television this time, but with the relatively new influence of cinema films. On this occasion, children between the ages of seven and seventeen were monitored closely during the night after spending a large part of the evening watching 'movies'. The evidence appeared to be conclusive: the films induced disturbed sleep, and the researchers advised caution over children's evening activities if sleep quality was to be preserved. What was perhaps more important, though, and was to become clear in later experiments, was the effect staying up late had on the *depth* of children's sleep. It seemed that the later they stayed up at night, the more difficult they were to wake up in the morning, and the more likely they were to be moody and have general attitude problems throughout the following day.

The same investigators followed with a series of experiments into the effects of insufficient sleep on young children, which highlighted a paradoxical effect of sleep loss. This was to be an extremely ambitious study for the time, involving almost 7,000 nightly observations in a large sample of seven- to eighteen-year-old children. Most of them were already following a rigid schedule of nine hours' sleep per night, imposed by a residential institution.

The first stage of the experiments involved delaying the children's bedtimes from the normal time of 9pm to midnight. They were then woken up as normal at 6am. This left them with, at best, six hours of sleep per night. During these late nights the children played games, read and talked to the experimenters. In the next phase of the experiment, all children followed an alternative schedule, in which they were allowed to go to bed at their normal time but were woken up three hours before normal, at 3am. Again this enforced a regime of just six hours of sleep per night.

Children from across the whole range of age groups took part. Even the very young children had no real difficulty with either staying up late or getting up early. This probably rings true for many parents who will know that, provided they are occupied, children can quite easily and happily go way beyond their normal bedtimes without complaint.

The problems only emerged during school time, when child-carers and teachers found that the children gradually became more difficult to handle as the series of short nights progressed. This was particularly the case for the seven-year-olds, who suffered the worst from their reduced sleep. The report described the children being argumentative and irritable, and having little regard for normal social rules of behaviour. In the end, the protocols were eventually abandoned, as it seemed clear that these children were not getting enough sleep, to the detriment of daytime behaviour.

How can we tell when children have had enough sleep? Does a nine-year-old need the same amount as a 13-year-old? The children themselves will almost definitely insist not. In the Renshaw study in the 1930s, it was noticed that when children stayed up later, their sleep would be more profound and that they would be more difficult to wake than during sleep after a more 'normal' night. This was a similar observation to that of 'recovery' sleep after lengthy periods of total sleep deprivation in young adults, in which the first few hours were also inordinately deep.

In children, tiredness, particularly in the early stages, is not always obvious from their appearance. Again, this was picked up in the Renshaw study, which described a paradoxical 'pseudo-freshness' in the young children as the night progressed. This can obviously be very misleading for parents, and lends supports to a child's claim of not really being ready for bed. Children become irrational and insistent; as the authors note, 'tired children are the ones who fight hardest not to go to bed'.

It is interesting that the overall tone of this report is very prescriptive, and not far removed from current concerns. Despite its taking place some time ago, the authors were already talking about the effects of reduced sleep for children and 'the unnatural conditions of modern life'. Aside from cinema films and late nights, this was also to be one of the first studies to establish that caffeine was not particularly conducive to peaceful sleep in children. At the time, it was common for American children to drink both tea and coffee without any appreciation of its capacity to interfere with sleep.

Teen years and beyond

One of the problems with encouraging children to maintain reasonable bedtimes is that it is often very difficult for children to accept that they are ready for sleep. This is particularly the case as they get older and begin to push for autonomy in determining their own behaviour patterns. Sleep can become a question of control at this stage – they may deny their own tiredness and fight sleep for as long as possible just to prove a point. Bedtimes are also habit-forming – even young children often become so used to an 11pm bedtime that shifting to something earlier is not easy. Despite your resolve as a parent to insist on an earlier bedtime, getting a child to sleep is another matter. It will take some determination to bring bedtimes forward by even an hour or so, so there is very little point in the occasional early night.

Sleep-related behavioural problems are often difficult to identify. Bad moods, irritability and lack of concentration soon become seen as part of the child's 'temperament'. But insufficient sleep will almost certainly affect mood and irritability, if only because of the discomfort of feeling tired in a situation (such as a classroom) which does not allow you to sleep.

Changes in sleep patterns in the teenage years are highly predictable and related to the additional pressures of biological and social change. For many children, the onset of puberty coincides with later bedtimes, difficulty in getting up in the morning and oversleeping at the weekends. Part-time work and a greater interest in social activities in the evening all push the teenager towards a more adult daily pattern of sleep and waketimes.

For some, the pressure of academic goals can also have a negative effect on sleep. Transitional periods between high school and university education have been identified as periods of risk, particularly in the USA, but also in other areas of the world where academic achievement is highly valued. For instance, a 1993 report of high-school children in Taiwan found that older teenage students slept for as little as seven hours on week nights[2]. Preparation for examinations or related school work were the most common reasons given by the students for cutting back on sleep. But the incentive to sleep more is not always immediately obvious – in this survey, grade levels were actually higher for those students sleeping less, even though they were more likely to experience problems with overwhelming sleepiness during the daytime.

It's nice to think that there is room for compromise between work and sleep, but whether this is always effective is open to debate. Coping strategies, such as napping during the day, sleeping longer at the weekend, and increased reliance on caffeinated drinks, such as tea, coffee and cola, are all apparent at this age. One wonders how far poor sleep contributes to the already stressful events during this period.

Worries about children's sleep

Sleep-walking and night terrors

About three per cent of all children sleep-walk, although most of them grow out of this habit by adulthood. Sleep-walking occurs during the deepest stage of sleep, Stage 4. The sleep-walker can give the impression of being awake because it seems that they are purposeful in their actions, and yet they are difficult to rouse and they do not respond to efforts to communicate with them. Children do not generally remember the episode by the next morning. Most instances of sleep-walking are fairly harmless and cause the child little concern.

Night terrors emanate from the same stage of sleep, usually during the first one to two hours of sleep. The child will often wake abruptly from a night terror with a piercing scream as if in pain or genuine danger, and may appear to be inconsolable for some time afterwards. It is of some comfort to the parent to realize that there is usually no memory of the events by morning. Stress and sleep deprivation following a series of late nights are thought to increase the likelihood of night terrors. Most children can expect to outgrow them.

Bed-wetting (enuresis)

It is, perhaps, ironic that one of the most widespread and distressing problems associated with children's sleep – wetting the bed – is the one for which parents are least likely to seek medical attention. The reasons for this are unclear, although for most children bed-wetting (or nocturnal enuresis, as it is described medically) will almost always sort itself out before adulthood. There is also the perception that many of the problems leading to bed-wetting are due to social rather than medical factors, such as poor training or emotionally unsettling family circumstances.

Most children are expected to sleep through the night without needing to empty the bladder by around three to four years of age, sometimes earlier. Although boys are more likely to have difficulty with this, bed-wetting also seems to run in families, suggesting at least a partial genetic component. It may be that for some families the problem is not recognized as such until the child reaches five or six years of age, perhaps when they start school and more child-like as opposed to infant behaviour is expected of them. At this point, there is also considerable pressure on the child to conform to the expectations of a larger social group, in which many of their new friends will no doubt have achieved all-night dryness without difficulty.

Unless a dry bed can be guaranteed every morning, there are obvious limitations for a child's social development: sleeping over with friends, taking part in school or scouting camps, and having friends stay over all rely on mastering control of the bladder during sleep. And yet it has been estimated that wetting the bed is a problem for approximately five per cent of all six-year-olds and that a small proportion of these may continue to do so throughout adulthood. In recent studies, it has been estimated that this affects about one in 200 adults on a regular basis.

In terms of a physiological explanation, the reasons for being unable to go through the night without emptying the bladder during sleep are complex.

A number of possibilities have been suggested, including reduced bladder capacity, failure to suppress or reduce urine production at night (this is normally expected as the child matures) and failure to signal a need to respond to a full bladder – ie some children simply do not wake, while others also need to empty their bladder during the night but are able to wake up and go to the bathroom. And yet these possibilities represent fairly recent developments in this field. Overnight EEG studies of children have failed to find any significant differences in actual sleep patterns for children who wet the bed, although the possibility that these children have genuine problems with waking to a full bladder cannot be discounted, particularly as anecdotal reports from parents describe their children as unusually difficult to wake.

However, despite the possibility of some underlying physiological explanation, the association between childhood enuresis and a range of social and environmental factors is also very convincing. There is evidence, for example, that children with relatively young parents are more likely to wet the bed regularly. Heavy-smoking parents, birth order (bed-wetting is less common in first-born or one-child families) and social class are also thought to be risk factors. Exactly how these factors influence the development of bladder control through the night has always been unclear. Even so, bed-wetting has traditionally been treated with a combination of behavioural rather than physiological measures, which serve to reinforce the idea that the problem stems from a combination of inadequate 'training' and insufficient will on the part of the child.

Treatments have typically involved using an alarmed mattress sensitive to moisture, in combination with a positive system of reinforcements, such as a star chart to record successful periods of 'dry' nights and including some target incentive or reward for improvements. Medics will also use diuretics, particularly in older children, to reduce urine flow and allow the child to have the satisfaction of a dry night. Taking a child for treatment is nearly always seen as a last resort on the part of the parents, and the vast majority of children are simply allowed to sort out the problem in their own time. However, the psychological impact of continued bed-wetting can be huge in terms of self-esteem, confidence and personal growth. As a ten-year-old, it may be no reassurance to know that you will almost definitely 'grow' out of it.

Chapter 8

'I never sleep'

From time to time, we hear reports of people who claim to have gone without sleep for years on end. A recent report in the British-based *Daily Telegraph* newspaper[1] described how a Vietnamese woman by the name of Nguyen Thi Le Hang went without sleep for over 30 years, despite being treated with conventional sleeping pills. In Cuba, a 53-year-old man by the name of Tomas Izquierdo complained of not having slept for over 40 years. His insomnia was later confirmed during a two-week stay in a sleep laboratory, during which it is claimed that he remained awake the whole time (although whether this had been the case for over 40 years is still debatable). In India, an 80-year-old man described how he hadn't slept at all for over 45 years.

These reports are popular in the press, although often difficult to verify and therefore treated with some degree of scepticism. It is also quite rare to hear of such extreme claims. Many people will describe how they are not getting nearly as much sleep as they would like, and education about expectations of sleep, particularly with increasing age, can help to alleviate some of these concerns. For a small fraction, though, the problem lies with being able to identify when sleep has actually happened. Unless we are aware of sleeping, the chances are that we will over-estimate how long we have been awake. This can often cause difficulties for the insomniac, who remains unconvinced even after being shown objective evidence of sleep-like EEG brain patterns taken during a laboratory assessment.

What does it feel like to be asleep?

With the exception, perhaps, of lucid dreaming (see Chapter 11), we usually remain oblivious to having slept until after the event, and even then we may have our doubts if it creeps up on us unexpectedly, or perhaps when it is embarrassing for us to admit. The same is true for waking up in the middle of the night, as brief awakenings, such as a trip to the bathroom, can often be forgotten by morning.

Although we have come to think of it as a simple process, falling asleep is rarely an all-or-nothing transition. We often conceptualize sleep as a 'shutting-down' process, and yet there is the paradoxical state of dreaming, in which the mind is extremely active. Furthermore, it is possible that many people actually sleep more than they realize. The sleeping state tends to suggest a general dampening of awareness of the mind's activities along with a reduction in sensitivity to internal and external stimulation. Usually, and in the right circumstances, sleep occurs spontaneously and with little conscious effort, although the individual has only a tenuous control over this process.

In insomniacs, for example, there is frequently a wide discrepancy between estimated sleep times and those observed under laboratory conditions. Often, one of the treatment priorities is to offer reassurance by convincing people that they have actually slept for a reasonable length of time. In order to understand why people find it difficult at times to recognize that they have been asleep, it is necessary to have a clearer picture of what the early period of sleep entails. A more thorough understanding of the mechanisms involved in the process of falling to sleep is not only important in the treatment of patients for whom these mechanisms seem to have broken down, but also to help prevent sleep in potentially hazardous situations, such as while driving or operating machinery. We know through casual observations that sleep can sometimes fool us. Intuitively we might expect to notice even a momentary loss of awareness, but under laboratory conditions there is evidence to suggest that most people need to be 'asleep' for about two minutes before they have a subjective experience of having 'slept'.

So how can we define 'sleep'? There are many levels to this and they may not always be in agreement, particularly around the boundaries of sleep and wakefulness. This can produce bizarre and often worrying effects – some of which are discussed in more detail in later chapters. During a state known as sleep paralysis, for example, the body is effectively immobilized, although the mind is active and there is conscious awareness similar to being awake, yet also very bizarre dream-like imagery. These borderline states suggest that the transition between sleep and wake is not always complete or clear cut (see Chapters 11 and 14).

Instead, we experience and observe sleep on many levels: in the way we react to the outside world and as a contrast to wake; in terms of the physiology of the body; and in our subjective awareness of it, ie the psychology of sleep. The integration of these three levels (illustrated in Fig 6 on page 107) produces what we know as being 'sound asleep'. In order to fall asleep, and experience it as such, it is necessary to maintain a delicate balance between these three levels.

Response to the outside world

Although we are apparently asleep, the brain is still actively monitoring and responding to events taking place in the outside world (but with a certain degree of filtering in order to preserve sleep). This allows the parent of a new-born child, for example, to ignore all other sounds but respond immediately to the unique cry of their infant in the middle of the night.

In light sleep, most people are still able to perform basic tasks set for them in the laboratory. This might include listening for a specific sound and react-ing as instructed, or waking at the sound of their name. Studies have also shown that it is quite common to incorporate events that are going on around us into a dream during sleep; these might include unfamiliar sounds or movements in the bedroom, or ideas transplanted by an experimenter whispering into the ear of a dreamer. During sleep talking, it is possible to encourage a response from somebody who appears to be sound asleep, even though that response may be jumbled and largely incoherent, suggesting that they are nevertheless processing incoming information on some level. Also, the findings of studies of noise pollution during the night indicate that the body responds to things going on around it, even though we may not con-sciously register this disturbance or have any specific memory of it.

Sensitivity to the outside world changes throughout the night, and will depend to a great extent on the stage of sleep, as well as the importance of the incoming information. As with the example of the baby crying, it seems that we are very selective over what we prefer to respond to – unless, of course, the level of interference is so great that we are no longer able to ignore it. Sensitivity also varies a great deal from one person to another, with some people appearing to be oblivious to almost any amount of commotion.

Sleep and the body

The body is said to be asleep at the point at which the EEG waveforms change to a distinguishable 'sleep' pattern. There is a widely adopted standard for identifying this pattern (see Chapter 3). Unless there is some underlying sleep disorder or an extreme urgency for sleep brought about through, say, staying up much later than usual, there is a fairly predictable chain of events from being wide awake through to deep sleep.

Under these circumstances, after turning off the lights and lying down, the first signs of sleep will begin to show within 20 minutes or so. Stage 1 sleep is preceded by a period of drowsiness; the muscles begin to relax and the eyes may roll upwards into the eye sockets. Heart and respiration slow down into a relaxed, regular pattern and brain activity begins to slow into a less erratic pattern. Alpha activity, indicative of quiet, restful wake, is gradually replaced by slower theta waveforms, as Stage 1 sleep develops. However, during this period, there is some waxing and waning between sleep and wake, before sleep can be said to be fully established. This is also a period in which we are easily disturbed and will respond without difficulty to things that happen around us, or on hearing something in which we are interested.

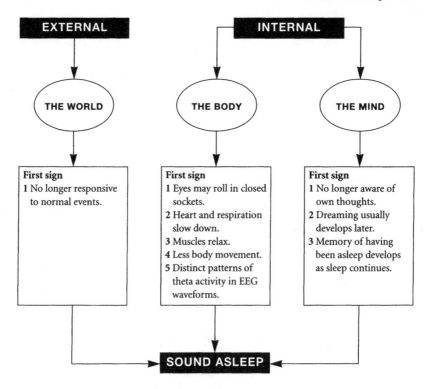

Fig 6 **Levels of sleep: from wake to light sleep.**

Most normal sleepers 'know' that they have slept only if sleep is allowed to progress to some depth, usually coincident with the appearance of Stage 2 waveforms in the EEG. If sleep continues, deeper Stages of 3 and 4 follow soon afterwards. However, reconciling the subjective experience with objective measures of sleep can be more difficult in certain cases.

Sleep and the mind

Even though the body may be going through all the right motions, if the mind is not willing then sleep is difficult. Worries about the day's events or future concerns all conspire to keep the mind active. Simply falling asleep, not matter how physically tired you are, can be almost impossible with the mind in this state. It is important to target these difficulties before any further problems develop, as insomnia is both caused by and causes stress and anxiety.

Many old-fashioned remedies suggest replacing mental activity with more benign thought processes – such as counting sheep, for example. Although not everybody is so easily pacified, this approach, or something like it, can help to preoccupy the mind in order to achieve sufficient mental relaxation for sleep to occur. In extreme cases, problems persist throughout the night as the mind continues to ruminate on negative ideas or thoughts during sleep. This can be very unsettling and may lead to the impression of having had little sleep by morning, or no real benefit from being asleep. For these reasons, it is important to resolve psychological problems as far as possible before going to bed, or at least to attempt to clear the mind and relax in preparation for sleep.

Falling asleep

Clearly, there is a wide range of conditional factors which serve to influence the potential for sleep, many of which were discussed in Chapter 5 in relation to the question of how much sleep we need. There is rarely a simple equation between factors to account for sleep on a particular occasion, as the properties of the body, the mind and the outside world and their influence on sleep are changing constantly. It is perhaps more useful to think of the transition between wake and sleep as a period of fluctuation, in which competing demands for staying awake determine the likelihood of continuous and uninterrupted sleep. At least partial closing down of both the outside and the inner worlds is essential in order to progress to sound sleep. Should problems arise, it is possible to target one or other of these areas and enhance the chances of sleep, although this may take some determination and effort as sleep difficulties quickly become habit-forming.

Under normal circumstances, the dominance of a particular factor is likely to be unremarkable, and it may only be in extreme circumstances, such as following an acute loss of sleep, that we can expect to fall asleep very quickly. The rest of the time we rely on a delicate balancing act, in which falling asleep, or simply being less awake, can be a drawn-out process. However, being asleep and knowing that we are asleep do not always coincide with each other.

Part 3

Sleep and the psyche

Chapter 9

An obsession with dreaming

I t's a fairly safe bet that we all dream for at least part of every night asleep, although our memory might tell us otherwise! On the face of it, most of our dreams are nonsense, comprised of disjointed, complex and unpredictable storylines. We are indiscriminate in allocating key roles to complete strangers, loose acquaintances, close friends or loved ones. Our waking relationships with those involved, no matter how intimate or long term, do not guarantee that they will behave 'in character' in our dreams. They can be transformed mid-dream and without warning in terms of appearance, mood and intentions. Nor is the plot constrained by natural laws of time and place, with frequent, unpredictable shifts taking place in pace and location.

At best, we wake with a sense of bemusement at the sudden reappearance of long-forgotten, apparently insignificant characters from our past. At worst, we wake feeling frightened and anxious. Of those dreams that are remembered on waking, their effect is usually transient, occupying our thoughts for no more than a few minutes at the start of the day. At the other extreme, a particularly disturbing dream can be difficult to shake off, leaving an unpleasant and lingering aftertaste throughout the day.

We engage in our dreams on many levels, from the intensely disturbing and bizarre dream in which we are the central character, to the less emotive, voyeuristic-style dream which demands only limited involvement. While the former is more likely to provoke basic, raw emotions, such as fear, pleasure and desire, in the voyeuristic dream our role is relatively impassive: we may be perplexed by the cryptic nature of events, but we are less anxious or concerned about them. Dreams also vary considerably in their abstractness – from, at one extreme, those which follow logical and realistic patterns of thought, governed by language and rationality, to the more surreal 'sensation'-type dream, which can leave nothing more than an overwhelming sense of gloom or anxiety without obvious focus.

A passion for dreams

Dreams are very much in vogue at the moment. The public demand for books, magazine articles or professional services offering to unravel the individual mysteries of our dreams is, apparently, endless. It is claimed that we now have the technology and the knowledge to make radical changes to our dream experience, by eliminating much of the spontaneity and unpredictable flow of the dream in preference for one in which we get to choose invited participants, location, duration and turn of events. Known as 'lucid' dreaming, this is an intriguing possibility for many people, who find the idea of being aware of the dream as it happens and acting with volition to influence the unfolding events preferable to the erratic, uncontrolled nature of everyday dreams. Advocates of lucid dreaming claim to have discovered an additional dimension to human experience, for which individual imagination is the only real limitation.

The possibility that we can have control over our thoughts, and even our actions, during sleep, contradicts an intuitive understanding of sleep, with obvious implications for legal and philosophical issues concerning questions of human agency and individual responsibility during sleep. Are we responsible for injury to others or ourselves if we are asleep at the time? Common sense suggests that to be responsible for our actions we need to be both aware of the event as it happens and in control of our actions. Until recently, neither of these conditions have been associated with sleep. Lucid dreaming opens up new possibilities of awareness during sleep and, as a result, it may be necessary to revise our understanding of what it is that we are capable of during sleep, and how responsible we are for any consequences. These issues will be discussed in greater depth in Chapter 13.

Dream recall as self-knowledge

For many people, one of the most intriguing aspects of dream investigations is the promise that through our dreams we are offered an insight into the workings of our inner self: the dream cannot lie! For some time now there has been a great deal of excitement about the prospect of getting to know ourselves through dreams which offer (the expert) access to a previously inaccessible subconscious life. We submit our dreams willingly and with pleasure to partners and friends, while unwittingly revealing their true nature only to the trained listener.

Over recent decades, we have witnessed the emergence of a large industry of dream-workers in response to this 'need' to know and, importantly, a willingness to talk about ourselves to others in order to achieve this end. Dream interpretation provides us with another layer of understanding through which we can achieve our ultimate goal of inner peace and fulfilment – knowledge of our psyche.

Does this willingness to explore publicly our most intimate and personal world reflect a more general shift in social structures and relations which, on the one hand, promotes individual happiness through self-knowledge, and on the other, sees the decline of organizations with have traditionally supported this very aim – the family, the close-knit neighbourhood, the church and so on? Nor is this urge towards self-disclosure limited to the world of dreams: there is now a more general demand for telling all in many areas of human life. From the wayward politician, sports personality or celebrity, who is granted public absolution through the media in exchange for a convincing display of 'self' exposure, to the prisoner who enhances parole opportunities through the process of admission, explanation and repentance, the modern-day 'confession' has taken on a unique position in our society.

Does the eagerness with which we submit our innermost thoughts to complete strangers, professional or otherwise, indicate a growing reliance on the belief that it is only through self-knowledge that we can achieve deep and lasting happiness? If so, this is an important development for many cultures where personal happiness is now considered vital to physical well-being. It follows that, as we become more comfortable and at ease with the idea of self-revelation, we expect to move closer to a state of enlightened liberation – hence the increasing range of opportunities for the expression of personal experiences, feelings and desires. The process of introspection, by which we look inwards and examine our thoughts and motivations, has become a daily part of public and private lives, from marriage guidance, family and personal therapy to the ritualistic displays of television chat shows, to the extent that a reluctance to do so is viewed as unusual.

Unhappiness is now the legitimate domain of the counsellor, such as a dream therapist, who provides a professional service, incorporating objectively determined scientific knowledge. As part of this scientific 'package', the dream provides an important tool for the analyst and is a central theme in many of the more popular attempts to understand the human psyche. In order to appreciate fully the value of this approach, we need to note a number of underlying assumptions regarding the role of the dream in a therapeutic context:

• The dream provides a pointer to the source of emotional and psychological difficulty.

• The dream relies on the 'language' of the subconscious, which can only be unravelled by the trained analyst.

• In dreams, reference to a traumatic experience is hardly ever direct.

• Our innermost concerns are actively repressed by the conscious mind and we are unaware of their significance while awake (although from time to time they may 'leak', as with a 'slip of the tongue').

• Recurring dreams are caused by long-standing, neglected anxieties or emotional conflicts.

• Dreams are extremely important: they act as a 'safety valve' through which psychological pressure is released by providing an opportunity to negotiate our most painful anxieties without distress.

Why do we dream?

The development of greater sophistication in the methods of the biological and psychological sciences has led to a diverse range of approaches to the question of why we dream. We can now 'decode' the dream at many levels, and are no longer limited to the subjective experience of what it is like to dream. Through brain-imaging techniques and EEG recordings, it is now possible to describe what is going on in the brain at a biochemical and elec-trophysical level during dreaming – to show which areas are active and which relatively inactive compared with when we are awake. Neuroscientists are able to redefine the concept of dreaming in terms of that which can be observed objectively. Contrast these developments with the psychodynamic explanation for dreaming outlined below, which relies extensively on indi-vidual memory and reconstruction of a dream.

However, no single approach has been able to produce a definitive expla-nation for the role of dreaming as a universal, everyday occurrence in modern life. In the following sections, these approaches are explored in greater depth by asking whether the experiential approach to dreaming has been seriously undermined by a more 'scientific' approach. Without dismiss-ing the contribution of neuroscientists in recent years, it seems that we are now much closer to understanding *how* we dream (where it takes place in the brain) than *why*.

The psychodynamic explanation

Popular dream theories have been influenced enormously by the psycho-dynamic movement, and in particular the theories developed by Sigmund Freud[1]. In a selective format, his ideas provide an accessible account of the cryptic nature of the dream, while also prioritizing the dream as central to human happiness. Freud alerted both public and scientific interest to the importance of dreams, and in doing so secured a place for the dream in modern science – or perhaps more specifically, the science of mental health.

Originally trained as a medical doctor, Freud developed his treatment for psychological distress within the context of his clinic in Vienna. His work met with considerable criticism from opponents who were reluctant to accept the possibility of meaningful mental activity during sleep, a condition otherwise understood to be a state of unconsciousness, lacking any level of brain engagement. In addition, his methods relied to a great extent on both a willingness and ability on the part of the patient to provide true and full accounts of a dream experience. There followed from this a significant level of subjective interpretation on the part of the practitioner. Within a short period, however, Freud's techniques were proving useful in dealing with the psychological trauma experienced by 'shell-shocked' soldiers returning from the front lines of World War I. This experience made many medical practitioners more sympathetic to Freudian theory.

These days, and with the recent experience of the Falklands and Gulf wars, there is nothing unusual in the idea that returning combat soldiers should depend on extensive counselling to deal with the emotional and psychological traumas of war, despite the fact that they may be physically unscathed. On this point, it is interesting to note that the anxiety dreams associated with combat have been shown to return 50 years later (see Chapter 4).

The psychodynamic approach is premised on the understanding that the mind is active in repressing memories, experiences, traumas and anxieties that we find too disturbing to confront. When emotional distress reaches acute levels, complete psychological breakdown can follow. Freud recognized that the intervention of the analyst depended on access to the source of this breakdown, and saw an opportunity to do just this by decoding the dream. Freud argued that we all share common types or elements of dreams, and that rather than being influenced solely by prevailing cultural values, certain dream themes are universal and can be traced back to early historical dream accounts or even across geographically distinct cultures.

Many current popular views of the dream borrow from Freud' s work, in particular the belief that the dream is an essential and natural part of every night and that it contributes towards stabilizing an otherwise fragile mental equilibrium. This view prioritizes the unconscious operations of the mind in dealing with events or concerns which are so disturbing or unsettling that we are not able to cope with them at the conscious level – hence the apparently meaningless code of dreams. By denying us direct access to the more disturbing aspects of our inner lives, the mind is protecting us from possible psychological trauma or breakdown. However, rather than bottle up all these concerns there is still an urgent need for them to be addressed and resolved, and this is precisely the role of the dream.

Problems arise when the mind is no longer able to cope with a particular event or trauma and the psyche becomes transfixed. Preoccupation, dread and recurring dreams are symptoms of this state. At this point, the psychological development of the individual is severely compromised and professional help is needed. Freud developed a technique known as psychoanalysis, through which he attempted to make sense of the nonsense of dreams by revealing the underlying thoughts, events or preoccupations responsible for a particular dream scenario.

If we accept this view of the dream then, barring problems, you might think that we should just let the mind get on with its work and sit back and enjoy the ride. Not so – the dream is seen by many as a direct route to self-knowledge and fulfilment.

Many of Freud' s original ideas have now become part of modern 'folklore' regarding the importance and interpretation of dreams and their relation to everyday life. In terms of historical significance, the work of Freud and the advent of psychoanalysis has had a profound effect on the popular conception of dreaming (see Chapter 2). In particular, his work placed a great deal of importance on and drew much attention to human sexuality, especially in relation to children, and its fragility in terms of pathological development.

Freud helped to establish the focus of dreams as latent, secretive and repressed. As a powerful technique for the extraction of the truth about dreams, psychoanalysis offers a means to self-discovery through the assumption that dreaming is essential to human functioning. In dealing with psychological disturbances, the psychoanalyst is equipped with the knowledge to understand the true meaning of the dream and assist the individual in resolving the central difficulties. However, the individual must first be convinced of and aspire to know the truth of the dream.

In this sense, Freud has made a substantial impact, not simply as the 'discoverer' of dreams, but as the driving force in making the idea of dream analysis more palatable to the individual, and the whole concept of the dream more amenable to scientific investigation. In particular, through the development of scientific methods of inquiry, language and interpretative expertise, it has been possible to produce calculable and documented information about the dream and to establish what is and is not 'normal'.

In working towards observable and universal rules of human behaviour, Freud aspired towards scientific rigour and emphasized the importance of control, method and generalizability. However, modern scientists are less keen on introspective techniques for understanding human behaviour, preferring instead to rely on that which can be seen and manipulated objectively – hence the focus on changes in the brain in order to explain the activity of the mind during sleep.

Despite this, Freudian theory has an enduring appeal at a popular level, largely because it offers an intuitive explanation for the way we have come to view our dreams. It also recognizes that we live as social animals, rather than as individual units explained as the sum of our brain activity. On the whole, many of us are happy with the idea that the mind is a complicated affair which will not reduce easily to a substance in a jar, and have come to expect explanations for human behaviour in terms of thoughts, drives and motivations rather than chemicals and brain matter. For this reason it is perhaps worth exploring Freud's work in more detail, bearing in mind that there are many alternative views on the role of the dream.

Wishful thinking

A central theme in Freud's work was that of the dream as a wish-fulfilment experience, in which we act out desires and impulses that we are unable to achieve during consciousness. In this respect, he found that many young children's dreams were startlingly transparent, in that they would often be a repetition of a particularly enjoyable event which had occurred during the previous day or a realization of events which they had been prevented from enjoying during the day. The bizarre and cryptic nature of the dream was understood not to emerge until such time as children became aware of certain taboos concerning their focus for pleasure. Freud linked this development with the onset of moral and ethical awareness. This relies on an understanding of basic divisions within the mind, which, according to Freud, have a direct and competitive influence over our conscious behaviours.

Freud described three powerful forces within the mind, the sum of which results in our unique personality or identity: the 'id', the 'ego' and the 'superego'. The id represents our most primitive, unrestrained drives and impulses and is drawn towards selfish pleasure. The superego represents our awareness of social and parental values and acts as a sort of social consciousness in overseeing our actions. This element of our personality only really becomes established as we begin to develop a sense of moral and ethical awareness. The ego acts as a governing body through which the demands of the id and the superego are managed.

While the id excites interest in self-serving activities, especially those of a sexual nature, the superego polices behaviours to ensure that these are acceptable within the prevailing norms of family or social life. As the individual is subjected to the increasing restraints imposed by the ego (under threat of guilt or anxiety if the forbidden behaviours being demanded by the id are actually carried out), there is increasing conflict between the two processes.

According to Freud, the dream is an essential route to resolving this conflict. As the child gets older there is a preoccupation with sexual interest and anxieties, especially in relation to parents, placing a greater pressure on the ego to transform these desires into acceptable social behaviour. As we become aware of the forbidden nature of these wishes, we explore the process by hiding their true nature from conscious awareness. At around this time, the conflict between id and superego invades the child's dreams and they begin to take on a more bizarre, cryptic form. In particular, we see the emergence of veiled references to sexual and taboo practices. The focus for this preoccupation is transformed into an unrecognizable state: for example, a father-figure may be represented as a dark, ominous entity, and so on.

Freud distinguished between 'manifest' and 'latent' dream content. 'Manifest' refers to the content of the dream as we experience it: the bizarre and unpredictable characters, shifts in plot, disruption to time, etc. He contrasted this with the 'latent' content of the dream, which refers to the underlying dream content: that coded content which contains hidden references to our innermost impulses, drives and emotional preoccupations. For the period, this was a relatively dramatic shift in thinking.

Freud was highly dismissive of suggestions that the source of dreams was external to the body – for example, spiritual or religious interventions – and ambivalent towards the view that dreams could be accounted for solely by the intrusion of bodily functions (eg gastric) into the dream state. Instead, he emphasized the importance of the dream as a psychological event generated solely from within an individual and contingent upon the operation of the subconscious.

For example, it was the subconscious which was responsible for the transition from latent to manifest dream content; this Freud termed 'dream work'. The reversal of this process was, in his view, achievable through psychoanalysis, during which the true meaning of the dream could be drawn out. Freud's aim was to offer analysts universal laws of association between symbols and underlying meaning, in order that they could make sense of the unintelligible connections between events and characters during dreams.

Dreaming and empirical science

We use the word 'empirical' to describe scientific investigations that prioritize describable, measurable, observable and controllable features. In that sense, the introspection of dream recall (allowing the discussion of inner thoughts and experiences) does not fall into the category of empirical observation. This was seen to be problematic by many scientists, including those interested in sleep, who wished to emphasize the scientific strengths of the psychological sciences. One way to get round this was to concentrate on features of the dream which could be measured more easily – for example, what happens to the brain, and the body, during dreaming?

Dreaming and REM sleep

The impetus for dream research was maintained during the 1950s and beyond by a number of landmark studies into the nature of brain activity during sleep. Since this point, many of the popular conceptions of the dream have been inconsistent with the available scientific knowledge. Although dreaming is still viewed by a significant number of researchers to be a fascinating and important area of scientific research, it does not feature on the contemporary scientific agenda to the same extent as in the first two decades following the initial discovery in the 1950s of the brain state attributed to dreaming[2].

This was made by two of the early pioneering sleep researchers, Aserinsky and Kleitman, who noticed that while their volunteers were asleep, at certain times of the night, and with predictable regularity, their eyes would flutter around in an apparently random fashion under closed lids. They described this as a period of 'rapid eye movement sleep', to be known as REM sleep, as distinct from the remainder of the sleep period when the eyes were still, to be known as non-REM or NREM sleep. It became obvious that the likelihood of reporting a dream experience after sleep involving rapid eye movements was very high, hence the assumption that REM sleep is synonymous with dreaming sleep (although subsequent research has questioned whether REM sleep is either a necessary or sufficient condition of dreaming as an experience).

Early laboratory-based studies of dreams prompted by the landmark discovery of REM sleep were not unsympathetic to Freud's ideas. While dream content provided access to the subconscious areas of the mind, further quantification of the brain's activity during dreaming was assumed, with some enthusiasm, to provide complementary information and to contribute towards an overall understanding of the dreaming process, with an explanation of the reason for dreaming as the ultimate goal.

Studies of REM sleep from the late 1950s onwards provided a fascinating insight into the activity of the brain and the body during this state. At this time, there was no problem with the assumed link between REM sleep and dreaming – hence introspective techniques for linking body with mind were popular. A number of assumptions were made:

• The transition from REM to NREM sleep follows a distinct cycle throughout the night. As we have more than one period of REM sleep each night, we must experience more than one dream period.

• Although we are sometimes left with the sensation of timelessness – as if the dream were over in a split second – dreams last for as long as the REM period. This is more likely to be minutes rather than seconds.

• This assumption is further supported by the finding that longer REM episodes tend to result in more complicated, lengthy dreams. It is likely that we actually dream in 'real time', and not a distorted version of time as our senses sometimes suggest.

Dreams as a consolidation of the day's events

One wonders if the content of a dream bears any resemblance to the more superficial aspects of a day's events. Even though dreams do not always bear a one-to-one resemblance to the things that have happened to us during the day, the tone of the dream can nevertheless reflect our current emotional status. Difficult and upsetting upheavals, such as divorce, bereavement or unemployment, are often accompanied by disturbing dreams and restless nights. Dreams can also remind us of long-forgotten events that still trouble us on some level. Traumatic experiences occasionally re-emerge during dreams many years later, as with the group of French soldiers from World War II whose dreams contained direct references to events which had occurred some 50 years previously (see Chapter 5). Dreams can also reflect concerns in anticipation of a forthcoming event, such as childbirth, a new job or a house move, and may act as a psychological prompt for us to address issues which we have been putting off.

Distinct rhythms in digestive activity throughout the night have been thought to influence the content of dreaming through body awareness during sleep, and many people avoid certain foods during the evening – usually high-fat products such as cheese – specifically because of the presumed links between this habit and disturbing dreams. It is also possible for a dream to be influenced by sounds from the environment. This can happen when the alarm is set to a radio station and a news item or programme topic becomes submerged in an ongoing dream. A similar thing can happen if we are spoken to or touched while we are dreaming.

There has been a great deal of interest in the content of dreams in relation to real experiences, with many attempts to infiltrate dreams by manipulating exposure to external factors. Scientists wanted to know which factors, if any, influenced the 'dream script' or whether this was simply determined by the random firing of insignificant, misplaced memories of past events and future plans.

Direct experimentation with daytime experiences and their influence on dreaming has produced some interesting findings. For example, watching highly stimulating video films before going to bed can have both an immediate and a delayed impact on dreaming, with references to the imagery or content of the film being present on the first night and then again one to two weeks later. In contrast, less provocative comedies or romances of the 'family viewing' type have less effect on dreaming, suggesting that we are not just going over things that have happened to us, but that this really is a time for dealing with unfinished emotional business. Disturbing films can also increase restlessness during the night, a fact that may be of particular concern with children whose television viewing is unmonitored (see Chapter 7). The belief that external events, particularly those with a high degree of emotional impact, are incorporated into our dreams is not inconsistent with the psychodynamic understanding of the role of the dream, which is to assimilate potentially distressing experience. Known as dream 'incorporation' studies, the finding of a dream 'lag' as the delay between exposure to material and its subsequent insertion into a dream scenario mirrors observations made by Freud. Note that there is nothing hidden or unusual in these associations, but at its simplest, dreaming reflects real and transparent fears and anxieties. If one of the functions of the dream lies in dealing with 'unfinished business' – ie coming to terms with things that upset us – then this certainly makes sense in the light of these findings.

Dreams as a 'safety valve'?

There is a more obvious parting of company between the psychodynamic and laboratory approaches to dreaming over the question of whether the dream acts as a psychological 'safety valve' in providing a nightly opportunity to 'let of steam'. If the safety valve theory is correct, and the dream really is essential (and not just useful) in reducing mental stress, we would predict that denied the opportunity to dream, the consequences would be traumatic.

The discovery of REM sleep meant that it was possible to put this theory to the test by using the EEG to monitor the electrical activity of the brain throughout whole nights of sleep. In this way, it is possible to follow the course of REM and NREM sleep and to eliminate, or at least dramatically reduce, the number of dreaming periods throughout the night by simply waking volunteers at the first sign of REM sleep. After a brief interval, the volunteer is then allowed to return to sleep. NREM sleep (presumed to be non-dreaming sleep) is still possible with this method, meaning that any effects on mood could not be attributed to profound sleepiness due to having had no sleep at all. Because volunteers are able to get a reasonable amount of sleep throughout the night, this method of REM deprivation can be repeated for days or even weeks on end.

It has been found, however, that as the nights go by following this technique, changes in the normal structure of sleep take place, with the first attempt to shift into REM sleep occurring earlier and earlier, and the number of attempted shifts also increasing. Volunteers are also described as more irritable and agitated by this disruption[3]. However, the effects are rarely extreme in terms of either mood, normal waking function, emotional stability or mental breakdown, providing little support for the psychodynamic argument that nightly dreaming is *essential* for mental health.

It is, of course, possible that these experiments never lasted long enough for the true effects of REM (dreaming) deprivation to emerge – perhaps we need weeks or even months without dreaming to invoke a serious psychological response. In support of this, it is noted that urgency for REM sleep increases as the experimental nights accumulate: volunteers are more difficult to wake and shift back into REM sleep at the first opportunity. Additionally, it may be that sufficient dreaming was actually achieved without the experimenters realizing, either during NREM sleep or during snippets of REM sleep, before the volunteer was fully awake.

It has been suggested that the difference between dream experiences in REM and NREM sleep are due to differences between the two brain hemispheres for these states. Specifically, following an awakening from REM sleep the dream account tends to be elaborate and detailed, prompting speculation concerning the role of the left hemisphere. In contrast, it has been suggested that the NREM dream is more dependent on functioning of the right hemisphere, as these dreams tend to be described in more abstract terms, to do with moods or sensations rather than concrete thoughts.

Bizarre, dream-like images also occur around sleep onset and waking up (hypnagogia and hypnopompia – see Chapter 3). Ordinarily, these events occur outside REM sleep – suggesting a different class of sleep-like brain activity. There are many well known examples of individuals inducing this sort of imagery in the belief that creativity and imagination thrive on the verge of consciousness. Is this dreaming?

REM sleep and depression

Over the years, experimenters have produced positive effects by manipulating the sleep of patients suffering from severe mood disorders. It became clear that many of these patients could enjoy an improved, more optimistic frame of mind simply by avoiding sleep! Patients who were kept up all night by taking part in individual or group activities on the ward were found to have a marked improvement in symptoms by the following day. As you might expect, there was a great deal of enthusiasm for this discovery, with many scientists keen to develop the technique as an alternative to existing treatments for mood disorders, which at the time were largely dependent on electro-convulsive treatment (ECT) or drugs, both of which involved undesirable after-effects.

Researchers were interested to know who could benefit, how long the effect lasted for, and how this was actually achieved in terms of brain mechanisms. It emerged that many depressed patients had an abnormal pattern of REM and NREM sleep through the night; typically, this showed as a shortened REM sleep latency (ie the first sign of REM occurred earlier than normal after sleep onset) and a longer first REM period, followed by intermittent periods of wakefulness and early-morning waking. These observations led researchers to speculate on the significance of REM sleep for depression.

It was pointed out that some anti-depressant drugs and ECT suppress REM sleep, and that perhaps this action has a significant role in their success. Unfortunately for the patients involved, many became depressed again at the first sign of sleep, prompting the suggestion of a mood-dampening substance released during sleep. To date no such substance has been identified, although the link between sleep deprivation and mood has remained an enigma for those involved in this research. In an odd way, these findings of a link between sleep and severe depression lend some support to the Freudian approach, which highlights the importance of dreaming for psychological functioning, although the relationship is not as we might expect.

The function of dreams

We are still a long way from a complete answer to the question of why we dream. The different approaches need not be mutually exclusive, but instead can provide different levels or layers of understanding for this intriguing experience: dream content may well be inspired by emotional states, but brain chemistry sets up the right conditions for the dream state.

In many ways, Freud rescued the dream and re-established it as an important, yet still mysterious, human experience. Modern cultures are keen to prioritize dreams, not (as in less 'advanced' societies) as a bridge between the mortal and immortal worlds, but as a route to self-knowledge. However, laboratory studies suggest that we can manage quite well without them.

Chapter 10

Premonitions and visitations

No matter how extraordinary the possibility, the idea that through our dreams we can have knowledge of events as they happen miles away from us, or have yet to happen in the future, has captivated the imagination for thousands of years. Although it flies in the face of our scientific understanding of the world, it is an enigma which has enduring appeal, sustained largely through individual and cultural beliefs, and undiminished by a failure to satisfy modern criteria of proof.

While the scientific approach has been preoccupied with the question of whether these phenomena actually exist and how to go about proving or disproving this, the reasons for wanting to believe that we might be able to predict events which go on to happen in some future time, to make psychical connections with loved ones at critical moments in their life, or to receive messages from them following death, is not high on the scientific agenda. Consequently, the current view is one of scepticism, with 'believers' presented as gullible and vulnerable people, lacking the facility to make an objective judgement about their experiences.

Take the 'precognitive' or premonition dream, for example, through which it is claimed the dreamer can witness events which have yet to happen. With this type of dream, the dreamer is privileged with knowledge that couldn't possibly be figured out through normal, rational means. This is not simply a belief that something *might* happen, but a powerful conviction that it *will* happen.

So what's wrong with the idea of premonitions during sleep? Quite simply, it does not fit with what we know about the world. The precognitive dream asks us to believe that some future event has already been decided at a higher level and that a select few can 'see' that event as it will inevitably occur in the future. This is not our experience of the world, in which we deal with a past (which we can remember), a present (which we are currently experiencing) and a future (which has yet to be decided and which we expect to have some input into shaping).

In westernized societies, the potential for determining the outcome of our lives is central not only to individual beliefs, but to the economic and social systems that we agree to take part in. The precognitive dream also presents serious difficulties for our basic understanding of the physical order of the world: no amount of true precognition is insignificant, and if precognitive dreams really do exist then this is a very important matter.

There is a certain intuitive appeal to the idea that, if we are capable of paranormal activities, then sleep (rather than wakefulness) would be the ideal time for this to happen, as the mind is less occupied with the rational world. Over the years, considerable effort has been put into trying to understand the nature of claims to paranormal activity, and particularly precognitive dreaming, during sleep. It is an area which has attracted all levels of investigation, including those claiming more rigorous scientific control.

The nature of precognitive dreams

Whatever your beliefs, support for the idea of precognitive dreams is very real, with the understanding that many people share a similar experience of it as a regular feature of their lives. The precognitive dream is described as a dream that includes details of an event which is later recognized as an actual event.

Accounts often emphasize the extraordinary sense of realism experienced during a precognitive dream – as if the person were watching the event unravel as an unseen bystander – as opposed to the generally messy and confusing dreams which we have come to expect. Descriptions of precognitive dreams often include some or all of the following features:
• Witnessing of an event that is not part of a memory.
• Knowing apparently trivial details of that event, either by seeing or hearing them.
• Witnessing death or injury to those involved, often close relatives but also strangers.
• It is also possible to view oneself taking part in an event.
• Although most precognitive dreams are thought to be intensely personal in focus, the best known are those dealing with a major public event, usually a catastrophic disaster.
• Experiencing a sense of dread or profound significance on waking.
• A confused understanding of the meaning of the dream, as the details can seem insignificant at the time,
• The same dream is sometimes repeated in minute detail, lending further support to the idea of its being extraordinary and important.

Many descriptions show that the precognitive dream is often not recognized as such until the associated event actually happens and becomes known publicly, at which point recollection of the dream can be extremely disturbing. With hindsight, the reference to an event can be startlingly clear, as the dreamer is reminded of specific details which could not be known through any other means. Although there is a natural tendency to look for possible coincidences to rule out the connection between the dream and the actual event, this latter point can be particularly unsettling.

On the other hand, actual proof of precognition is difficult to achieve. Researchers usually look for some evidence that the dream has been described to a reliable witness (or preferably more than one) *before* the event transpires and then only if similarities with the actual event are sufficiently convincing.

As with all dreams, memory of the content fades rapidly on waking. Apparently, the best way to save this memory is to write down as much about the dream as you can or describe it to somebody else, as soon as possible. Of course, most people are wary of attaching too much significance to their dreams and may be shy about being seen to take them too seriously. There is also a reluctance to appear unusual or simply attention-seeking on the basis of a dream. However, it is hard to believe that only people sympathetic to the idea of precognition during dreaming will be privileged with these experiences, and it may well be that most of these dreams, whatever their foundation, go unreported. (Contrast this with the attitudes of just 60 years ago, when publication of these claims was quite common. The British-based journal, *Proceedings for the Society for Psychical Research*, reported over 350 such cases in the first 50 years of its existence).

As it is generally claimed that events forecast in dreams occur within hours or days of the dream experience, the chances of having some influence over the outcome of these events are remote. Of course, this is a double bind situation as, at best, the claim to have influenced disaster as a direct result of acting on the predictions made during a dream (by persuading somebody to make alternative travel arrangements, for example) is nearly always going to be supported by a non-event. The exception to this is with an accident or disaster on a larger scale.

Experimental proof

It is not uncommon in the aftermath of a major public disaster, such as a plane crash, earthquake or accident at sea, for people to come forward with claims of having prior knowledge of the event during a dream or trance-like state. Many will see this as a particularly distasteful yet inevitable consequence of public access to tragedy on such a large scale. Consequently, these claims, although given a significant amount of attention in the popular press, are likely to be met with a great deal of scepticism and disbelief.

Having said that, there have been a number of attempts to catalogue and assess claims to precognitive dreams in relation to major disasters. Perhaps the best-known investigation of this type took place following the Aberfan disaster in Wales. On Friday 21 October 1966, shortly after the start of the school day, a mountain of coal residue shifted and slid down into the small

Welsh mining village, with devastating consequences. The village school was worst hit, resulting in the loss of 144 lives, including 128 schoolchildren. Within hours, and while efforts to dig out survivors were still going on, news of the tragedy was relayed throughout the world.

A British consultant psychiatrist by the name of John Barker asked whether there had been any forewarning of this event in the form of precognitive insights through dreaming or otherwise. In collaboration with the London *Evening Standard* newspaper, Dr Barker made the unusual request of appealing for individuals who believed they may have had a premonition of this event to contact him. This appeal was initially published seven days after the tragedy, with further mention in the other national and what Barker described as the 'psychic' press to follow. The appeal attracted over 76 replies in all, 36 of which made direct reference to a dream understood by the respondent to be a clear prediction of the disaster. Barker followed up those responses considered by him to be most convincing and reported his findings in the *Journal of the Society for Psychical Research* the following year[1].

Barker was particularly interested in 24 cases, basing this view on the number of features included in the premonition which were in common with the actual event, and whether or not the person had recounted their dream to reliable witnesses before the event occurred.

A substantial number of respondents recalled dreams involving children in distress, overwhelming or threatening images of blackness, and the sensation of suffocation. References to specifics were truly amazing, with some claiming to have dreamed of the town Aberfan, a Welsh miner, a communal graveyard, or a school building. Most premonitions were experienced within a day or so, or more likely just a few hours, before the actual event; however, the timing was corroborated by an outside source in only a relatively few cases. One case in particular attracted Barker's attention: that of a middle-aged woman who described her 'vision' of a mountain of coal sliding down on to a Welsh school – an experience she had apparently discussed with at least seven adult friends no less than 24 hours before the tragedy. In describing this vision, she recalled details which later bore startling similarities to the actual event, details which, according to Barker, she could not possibly have inferred without some degree of prior knowledge from whatever source. For example, the woman claimed to recognize from her vision a young survivor featured as part of the immediate news coverage. Although not strictly a dream premonition, Barker claimed this as one of the more impressive instances of prior knowledge.

In another example, a grandmother woke from her dream on the morning of the disaster with intense anxiety concerning her two young grandchildren. She had dreamed of a schoolroom in which children were trapped and struggling to breathe. On waking, her feeling of dread was so great that she spoke about it with adults at least two hours before the disaster.

For the individuals involved, the timing of their dreams and the nature of the tragedy is likely to have been profoundly unsettling. How can we explain Barker's findings? Well, as Barker himself pointed out, at the time of the accident the population of Great Britain alone was in excess of 50 million people. (This is, very loosely, the approximate number of people exposed to the advertising campaign in the *Evening Standard*.) We are reasonably sure that nearly everybody has at least one or two dream events each night, although we remember only a fraction of them. The possibility that 36 out of a total of 50 million people experience a dream, in fairly loose terms about children and large, dark mountains, is not particularly surprising, until it begins to take on the significance of such a highly publicized and shocking event as the Aberfan tragedy. Take any loose, random combination of characters and settings such as this, and the chances are that somebody is going to dream about them somewhere in a nation which experiences, on average, 100 million dreams per night.

This offers a plausible account, and suggests that we can expect pretty much all major public events which are both unexpected and devastating in nature to be followed by a small number of genuine claims from individuals who have experienced so much coincidence between a recent dream and the actual event that it has had a profound and disturbing effect upon them. Whether or not this is truly precognitive, in the sense that the two events are associated at some higher level, or mere coincidence is difficult to say – it may simply be that they had the misfortune of having the wrong dream at the wrong time.

In the case of the Aberfan disaster, we do not have to look too far into the general context surrounding this event for many of the apparently significant features of the reported dreams to be explainable in other ways – in which case, their incidence as a dream focus is not quite so surprising as we are led to believe.

• Anxiety for children is universal: concerns for their safety are an ongoing worry, especially in women.
• Images of blackness or darkness: there are obvious associations here with mountains of coal, but this imagery may also be symbolic of a more general fear of any kind of oppressive force.
• Specific reference to miners and the Welsh nationality: at the time of the tragedy the country was in considerable economic turmoil. The Labour Party conference had taken place just weeks before and the national press was dominated by daily accounts of industrial crisis, disagreements between unions and management, and strike threats. With the onset of winter, there would undoubtedly be worry about a repetition of the energy crises, strikes and power cuts of the previous winter. It is perhaps not surprising to find references to these concerns (in the form of key workers or coal-producing areas) in people's dreams.

Can we explain Barker's findings as unfortunate coincidence (36 out of 100 million)? Against this possibility, there are a number of specific references that seem to be truly remarkable – for example, dreaming the name Aberfan, or recognizing the face of a child survivor in a news report.

What is certain, however, is that most people within the newspaper advertisement circulation either didn't dream about the disaster, or were not willing to come forward and admit that they did. Of those who volunteered their experiences, many claimed that this was not their first experience of precognitive dreaming or 'knowing' about an event before it happened. A number of mediums, or what may be considered to be individuals 'sensitive' to these events, contributed to Barker's report. Most admitted having precognitive knowledge of other well-known events, including President Kennedy's assassination. This throws up a couple of possibilities;

• It takes a certain quality to be able to experience precognitive events; not all of us have it.

• It takes a certain quality to be able to believe in precognitive events when we have no direct proof other than subjective experience; not all of us have it.

A large majority of the accounts given were not corroborated by statements from friends or relatives who could confirm that the individual had disclosed details of the dream or vision prior to the event. In the absence of this supporting evidence, Barker relied to a great extent on his own intuition regarding the validity of the claims. This is not to suggest that these people were out to mislead him: in Barker's view, and after face-to-face interviews with many of them, they could be considered to be highly reliable witnesses. Most were women or girls who lived some distance from Aberfan and who were not personally affected by the tragedy outside their dream experience. He points out that he had no good reason to think that they were anything but sincere, or that they suffered any underlying neurotic state which predisposed them to delusions of this kind.

It seems clear that Barker was enthusiastic about further work in this area and that he saw great potential in harnessing the power of the precognitive dream. He implied that a greater understanding of this phenomenon could have enormous implications on a life-saving scale. Barker later went on to establish the British Premonitions Bureau in 1967, through which individuals were invited to contribute their own experiences of precognition, during dreaming or otherwise. The aim of this organization was to establish defensible records of dream premonitions before the predicted event actually happened, and possibly to provide an early-warning agency, especially where a large number of independent respondents claimed to have dreamed about the same event.

It makes you wonder why the subject of the precognitive dream is invariably one of doom and gloom. While people have claimed to have had blinding insight during a dream, or for brilliant ideas to jump out at them, these can usually be explained as acts of subconscious deductive reasoning (and have accounted for a number of significant scientific discoveries – see Chapter 2). But these ideas were already in the person's head at the time of the dream – sleep merely facilitated their development. To actually know something which can be turned to your advantage but which you couldn't possible expect to know through natural means – such as the winner of the 2.30 at Ascot – is another question entirely, and examples are usually limited to folk stories or drama. In fact, it seems that precognition during sleep almost invariably focuses on bad news.

Other visitations during sleep

There are many anecdotal accounts describing night-time visits, during a dream or following a sudden awakening, by a person who is later reported to have died. This person is usually a relative or a loved one and the time of their death coincides almost exactly with their visionary appearance.

There are no rational explanations for these events; usually they are not strictly precognitive and therefore there is little opportunity to act upon them. Instead, they are more likely to be described as telepathic events. So why so many at night? Sceptics might suggest that this is a period when we are most open to unusual experiences such as these. On the other hand, most people die at night, and as the coincidence between the timing of the vision and actual death is generally quite strong, the timing makes an awful lot of sense.

Researchers have found a clear link between sensitivity to these events and a more general willingness to believe in the paranormal. Nevertheless, nowadays 'believers' may be reluctant to discuss their ideas openly for fear of ridicule or of creating the 'wrong' impression. This has not always been the case, although there has always been some conflict in deciding where the dream exists. Is it as an event located firmly in the head – ie as a product of the imagination – or are we reduced during dreaming to a state more receptive to events outside the body that are not easily explained by modern scientific methods? This includes the projection of knowledge between dimensions, whether that includes past or future, dead or undead.

Precognitive dreaming and an alternative 'reality'

In 1927, J. Dunne published what was to become a classic study of precognitive dreaming – *An Experiment with Time*[2] – in which he described being struck with the realization that many of his dreams contained flashes from both his past and his future life. As you can imagine, this book caused quite a stir, even for the time, and is, in fact, still the focus of much debate among contemporary researchers.

Dunne was convinced that there was something odd about his dreams, following one particular incident in which his dream revolved around a disagreement over the precise time. In the dream, he was convinced that it was 4.30 in the afternoon, and when he awoke shortly afterwards he went to check the time on his watch. Finding that it wasn't on his wrist where he expected it to be, he eventually spotted it on a bedroom cabinet. The watch had stopped with the hands set at precisely 4.30. As this was a pre-digital watch, there would obviously be no way of knowing whether this referred to 4.30 in the early morning or afternoon.

Being a rational man, Dunne decided that, while it was impossible for him to read his watch face from a distance and behind closed eyelids, it was more likely that his watch had stopped at 4.30 that afternoon and that he had simply forgotten this. At the time he made no guess as to the actual time, but simply wound his watch to get it going again. He then went back to bed and slept on until morning when, to his surprise, he found that the watch was only a few minutes out. This suggested that he had indeed woken at 4.30am, ie at the same time as that indicated by the watch, even though it had stopped. The fact that he had achieved this without any external clues as to the exact time was a puzzle to him, especially as this particular time was a strong feature of the dream which had prompted him to awaken.

Perhaps Dunne had noticed the absence of ticking at the exact moment the watch wound down? We should not discount this possibility, as some people are particularly adept at keeping track of the time throughout their sleep, usually through an awareness of subtle but predictable changes in environmental noise, light and so on during the night. We should also be a little suspicious of such recollections, simply because awakenings during the night are not well remembered the following morning. We really need to be awake for at least one to two minutes before we have any recollection of being awake at all, and even then our memory for details will be vague. Is it possible that this wasn't Dunne's only awakening during that night, and that perhaps he had walked over to his watch a few minutes beforehand?

Nevertheless, Dunne was sufficiently intrigued by this experience to go on to monitor his dreams in great depth for the presence of further anomalies. So convinced was he by the results of his own investigations, that he developed an experimental protocol which he claimed would allow every individual access to their own dream potential. A central theme in his book is that precognitive dreams are not limited to a privileged few 'sensitive' people, as was previously believed; instead, Dunne argues that everybody has them, even though they may be ignorant of this fact.

Another reason that Dunne's book caused quite a stir was that it challenged the notion that time itself exists along a continuum, ie that we have a definite past, present and future. Dunne suggested an alternative view of the concept of time in order to explain his frequent insights into the future during dreams. At its simplest, Dunne suggested that past, present and future exist as one, and that we only understand it as a series of events because our brain organizes it this way. During sleep, the constraints of rationality and logic are lifted and our perception of time is no longer subject to the same rules of our waking existence. Hence we dream not only of past and current events, but also of events which we have yet to experience as part of our future, but which nevertheless already exist at the time of the dream.

This theory provided a direct challenge to the foundations of modern science by suggesting that (1) the future already exists and that (2) we can have access to it. From the outset, the idea of such a state seems unimaginable: if the future already exists, then what about causal relationships between events? Nearly all scientific endeavours have been geared towards describing, manipulating, predicting and ultimately controlling causality between entities.

Detecting precognitive dreams

Dunne provided extensive details of his early dream experiences through which he was alerted to the possibility of knowing the future. On first reading, it is hard not to be convinced by his claims to prior knowledge of a number of large-scale natural and man-made disasters. The fact that many of his precognitive dreams also involved mundane issues supported his belief that this type of dreaming was a natural, regular event rather than something unusual. With that in mind, he saw every dream as an opportunity to establish links with his waking experience.

Following initial observations of his own precognitive skills, Dunne went on to recruit a small number of acquaintances, mainly from friends and family members, who were willing to subject themselves to his methods of dream recording and analysis. He instructed them in a daily routine of extensive recording of all dreams on waking. Before sleep each night, they were expected to examine all dream accounts from up to 14 days previously and to judge each of them with respect to their similarity with the actual events throughout the current day.

All in all, Dunne presents an impressive account in which each of his volunteers is introduced to the precognitive nature of their own dreams – a feature which they had previously overlooked, but which, according to Dunne, they were eventually convinced of.

He was also fanatical in recording his own dreams, and advocated a strict regime for his readers who were interested in following suit. This included keeping a pen and paper next to the bed and, on the first instant of waking, writing down, with as much detail as possible, everything that could be remembered about the dreams which had taken place during the night. Dunne also gave advice on how not to lose the dream at the instant of consciousness due to its fragile and ephemeral nature. Rather than waste time on describing specifics in full, he recommended noting down *key words* which could be used to trigger vivid images related to the dream. In this way the dream could be rehearsed soon after waking, and the memory for it reinforced.

So remarkable were Dunne's claims that they attracted the attention of the British Society for Psychical Research, a group formed towards the end of the nineteenth century with the explicit aim of investigating paranormal phenomena through scientific means. Many eminent scholars of the time, in addition to lay members, were attracted to such ideals. Dunne's methods for discovering the precognitive nature of dreams were examined by Theodore Besterman on behalf of the Society and his findings were published in their journal in 1933[3].

Besterman attempted to replicate Dunne's findings by adopting 'to the letter' his method of dream recall and analysis outlined in *An Experiment with Time*. It had been intended originally that Dunne himself would co-operate with this investigation by working closely with Besterman throughout. However, it is clear from the disclaimer printed at the beginning of Besterman's report that the two men eventually parted company on a number of issues. Not least of these was Dunne's disappointment with the overall findings, and his claim that the reason for this was due largely to the inadequacy of instructions given to the volunteers willing to record their dreams for the purpose of the study. Even so, Besterman's report was not entirely dismissive of Dunne's claims.

An elaborate experiment was devised whereby volunteers were requested to make detailed notes of their dream recollections immediately on waking each morning. They were discouraged from spending too much time in trying to make sense of the dreams at this stage, but were to concentrate on including all details, no matter how irrelevant they might seem at the time. The dream report was then to be sealed in an envelope for delivery to the offices of the Society. It was impressed upon the volunteers that they were to complete this exercise before having any contact with the outside world through either the newspapers or by opening their mail. The original idea was that this would continue for a period of up to three weeks; however, in reality not all volunteers were able to produce a dream account on every morning of this period.

In addition to writing down their nightly dreams, volunteers were also asked to reflect on the events of their daily activities throughout this period and to make careful notes of any similarity between events as they unfolded during the day and their most recent dreams. These notes were then submitted to the investigators to be assessed in terms of a genuine precognitive relationship.

The first attempt at this involved a small group of middle-aged volunteers. At the time of the study there was perhaps less concern than nowadays about introducing bias into experiments relying on introspective techniques. The fact that these volunteers were all members of the Society for Psychical Research, and would probably hold strong views on the issues under investigation, was not seen as problematic. However, this attempt yielded little success, even though about one-third of those taking part made some connection between dreams and actual future events. On examination, the author concluded that only two out of a total 265 reported dreams were found to have sufficient similarity to subsequent events to suggest a case for precognition. He also went on to add that the trivial nature of the events involved in these two cases did not provide impressive support for this.

In one case, the volunteer recalled going to the cinema to watch a film about a yacht race and recognizing details of the layout of the boats on the screen from those 'seen' as part of a recent dream. From the details included in the published report, the degree of similarity between dream and event is not strong. Nor is there any discussion of whether the volunteer was involved in these types of activity as a hobby, or of any other circumstances (eg anticipation of a well publicized film) which might have led him to his dream before viewing the film. In this case, the association does not seem particularly remarkable.

What seems to have been overlooked in these early studies is the extent to which being involved, and focusing to an excessive degree on the content of one's dreams, is likely to influence behaviour, particularly as volunteers were asked to be on their guard for connections between their dreams and the things that happened to them during the day. This seems to ignore the fact that many of our experiences are brought about because we are able to act with a certain degree of volition and choice in the things that we do. For example, a dream about boats might encourage a trip to the cinema to watch a film about boats, even at a subconscious level, rather than predict it.

In the second case, the volunteer described how he dreamed of receiving an official letter through the mail, the night before one actually arrived. The letter was good news, which had apparently been anticipated for some time, so perhaps this dream was simply wishful thinking prompted by an event that was due any day.

At this point, Dunne was invited to comment on the predominantly negative findings, and he suggested that the age of those involved may have been a factor working against efforts to recognize connections between dreams and later events. In a second study, Besterman used young undergraduates from Oxford University. From an original sample of over 140 submitted dreams, he concluded that, at best, only two showed good signs of a precognitive element, but were not 'conclusive' evidence for it. Besterman's overall conclusions suggested that although he could not reject the idea of precognitive dreaming altogether, neither was he able to find strong evidence in favour of this possibility.

Possible explanations

Coincidence or reality?

Despite the many attempts to refute the possibility of precognitive dreaming, the belief in their existences is very real for whole sections of the population. So how can we explain the precognitive dream?

It may be possible to dream about something which later goes on to bear a disturbing resemblance to actual events; however, the sceptic will often look for another, perhaps simpler, explanation. Is the dreamer simply playing out a subconscious concern or fear for an event which has real risks, even though they may be unaware of this at the conscious level? Is the focus of their dream explainable in terms of anxiety, guilt or some other motivating factor? For example, if we have elderly parents or grandparents, then it is understandable that we should be sensitive to their increasing vulnerability. We may have real fears for their impending death or ill-health which we prefer to channel through the subconscious activity of dreaming. Dreams can also remind us of anxieties for ourselves which, more often than not, are brought about when the risk of an event occurring is high.

There is a well-known report in which President Abraham Lincoln had a premonition of his own death during a dream. He described being woken from his bed to the sound of sobbing from the rooms below. When he went to explore the origins of these sounds, he came across a crowded room in which its occupants were gathered around an elaborate coffin. On moving closer, Lincoln saw himself in the coffin. He later recounted this dream to no less than three people, and told how it had disturbed him so much that he had hardly slept for the rest of the night. Ten days later Lincoln was fatally wounded in an assassination attempt at a Washington Theatre.

On the night of the dream, Lincoln had been up late on important war business. After eventually going to bed, he remembered being asleep just minutes before the start of the dream. This seems rather misplaced for dream mentation of this sort and may well have been a hypnopompic experience rather than a REM dream (see Chapter 11). In addition, the dream starts in a very life-like style, with Lincoln lying on his own bed, listening to the sounds of sobbing from the rooms downstairs. By all accounts, the layout of the house in his dream (the White House) was familiar to his waking reality.

Was this a precognitive dream? By virtue of its timing, that would seem to be the case. However, unlike with many precognitive dream reports, there were no specific references or details given of the impending event. It is normal when dreams are associated with actual events for there to be some remarkable overlap in detail – we might have expected a veiled allusion to the assassination attempt, a gun, a theatre, the house across the road where he spent his final night fatally wounded. Instead, this dream focused on the aftermath of the event, and provided a very general account of a presidential funeral. The absence of more specific detail, or at least none recalled, might suggest that this was an anxiety dream about death in general rather than a precognitive dream about a specific event. After all, this was a man who had stayed up late waiting for important life-and-death news from the front line of battle.

Subconscious leaks?

The realization of a worry or concern that is playing on the back of our mind may find an opportunity to show itself during dreaming. Consequently, if that event later comes true it need not necessarily be evidence of precognition, but an illustration of how insightful the subconscious mind can be.

This argument has been put forward in the case of dreams about failing businesses, bankruptcies or other financial concerns, which the conscious mind may be reluctant to admit. It is also possible that the subconscious has greater insight into the condition of the body and is able to indicate genuine cause for concern, which may be unnoticed at the time of the dream but which later manifests as illness or disease.

An awareness of subtle changes in the environment also comes into this category: for example, changes in weather conditions such as temperature, humidity, or atmospheric pressure. Familiar engine noises, or the movement of physical structures to produce house noises, can alert the individual at a subconscious level to unfamiliar conditions, which are then incorporated into an anxiety-type dream. This is an accurate dream of a warranted concern raised by an acute sensitivity of which we are unlikely to be aware. When the dreamed event – a hurricane, storm, mechanical failure, roof collapsing – is actually realized, the dream is assumed to be precognitive because of the delay in confirming to the conscious mind what is already known at a subconscious level.

There have also been a number of attempts to link paranormal activity with the physical properties of the earth, particularly the role of geomagnetic activity. This research was conducted in the 1970s and 1980s under the assumption that external influences, such as fluctuations in the earth's magnetic forces, could somehow distort our subjective experience, including dreaming[4]. How this might be achieved – eg through altering chemical processes within the brain – is largely speculative. However, it offers an apparently plausible explanation for the belief that we might have had a dream which is quite different from our usual experience. Note in particular that, in contrast to 'normal' dreaming, the precognitive dream is more often than not understood to offer a literal representation of the forthcoming events, ie you see the events of a plane crash or earthquake almost exactly as it will happen. We do not normally expect to dream with such realism and this might explain why precognitive dreamers often wake up with the sense that they have had an 'extraordinary' dream.

Recognition through hindsight?

The mind has a remarkable capacity for clouding dreams, rendering their content meaningless and confusing. It is natural for us to try to resolve this confusion by reorganizing our dreams into some form of meaningful pattern. It is possible that, with the benefit of hindsight, the associations we make with real-life, often disturbing events may be overstated. Not only that, but we are apt to dismiss features of our dreams which do not readily lend themselves to the emerging picture. With rehearsal and fading recollection, our 'memory' of the dream is likely to move further and further away from the actual dream. There is also the problem of further embellishment from witnessing the aftermath of an event, often in minute detail, through the ongoing media reports, which invariably include images and eyewitness testimonies from the actual scene.

With all these problems likely to undermine claims to having 'seen' an event in a dream before it happened, it is perhaps not surprising that most people will dismiss this as nothing more than a vague association fuelled by coincidence and a taste for the macabre.

Premonitions with a happy ending

From time to time, we hear of people who have experienced 'near-miss' involvement in major accidents or tragedies. For every high-profile disaster resulting in the death of large numbers of individuals, there are people who came within a hair's breadth of being involved, often from nothing more than a last-minute change of heart in following through travel plans or going in to work. For these people, it is understandable that they would want to explain the awfulness of such an experience and the reasons for their narrow escape in some other way than sheer fluke. And yet few people have come forward who believe that their narrow escape was due to prior knowledge of the impending disaster, either through their own dreams or through those of a friend or loved one.

One interesting angle on this was taken in America in the 1950s by examining the passenger records in the period immediately prior to train crashes with high fatalities[5]. A distinct fall in passenger bookings on crash days (which could not be explained in terms of normal fluctuations) was found, as compared with the number of passengers travelling on the same schedule during previous weeks. Is it possible that this relates to some form of prior knowledge, even as just a hunch?

Even if this were true, it is difficult to imagine who would willingly take notice of such a hunch, however. Notwithstanding the objections to verifying precognition outlined earlier, there is a well-known story concerning a businessman who, having booked his passage on the *Titanic*, would only change his ticket for genuine business reasons despite the fact that he had a strong (and totally out of character) precognitive dream warning him against making the journey.

Who believes in the precognitive dream? It has been suggested that the sort of person who is more likely to take these experiences seriously has deep-felt concerns about their ability to either control or predict their life, and that beliefs in the paranormal act as a sort of protective mechanism against these anxieties. This seems rather a simplistic assumption to make, however, and many of the surveys of 'believers' show that they cover a broad spectrum of personality types. This is particularly the case for the 'out-of-body' experience (see Chapter 11).

Failed premonitions

As with the story of the boy 'crying wolf', it is difficult to know which warnings of impending disaster are genuine when recent history suggests that most can safely be ignored. This was a problem experienced by the two major attempts to record and isolate genuine cases of precognition. The first, already mentioned, was the establishment by Barker of the British Premonitions Bureau in 1967, followed shortly by the initiation of a New York agency known as the Central Premonitions Agency. One of the main aims in setting up these organizations was to provide an 'official' record of claims to precognition, rather than to rely on the anecdotal evidence of friends, relatives and other witnesses whose credibility was never beyond doubt.

A number of interesting issues emerged. Over a six-year period, the British Premonitions Agency took no less than 1,200 calls reporting premonitions. Of these, the vast majority could not be linked with an actual event. There were one or two exceptions, but these cases stemmed from a small group of individuals who made regular claims to dreams of this kind. This is an interesting point because, without assessing the validity of the dreams in themselves, it does suggest that this phenomenon is restricted to a limited number of people who are special in some way, rather than being a universal trait.

Both agencies were eventually closed after failing to produce unequivocal evidence of precognition – and, it should be added, failing to avert a single potentially catastrophic event through their activities. This raises questions concerning the nature of the future. Is the future fixed, in which case precognitive dreams are simply voyeuristic 'tasters'? Or is what is seen just one of a number of possible outcomes? The quest of organizations such as these assume the latter, and that there is room for intervention, given adequate warning.

Nowadays, there are still a number of self-organized groups keen to monitor claims to precognitive events along similar lines to their predecessors.

Details of the activities of these groups were largely confined to specialist magazines until recently, when interest in these issues was revitalized as part of a more general enthusiasm for science fiction and the paranormal in the 1980s and 1990s, especially among Internet users.

A subjective reality

Given the various possibilities outlined in this chapter, it seems very likely that reports of the incidence of precognitive dreams are underestimated, as a result of a more general prejudice against the idea of the paranormal. And yet, subjectively, these experiences are genuine for many people and can have a powerful effect on their lives.

Chapter 11

Where are we when we sleep?

Flying and falling dreams are extremely common, and occur more often at times of stress or high anxiety. Occasionally we wake from these dreams with a sudden jerk, as if we really are falling off the building, cliff or mountain seen in our dream. This coincidence between physical and dream imagery is common during the early stages of sleep, perhaps when we drift unexpectedly into sleep for just a few minutes. Despite physical sensations filtering through into the early fragments of consciousness, that momentary sensation of weightlessness, as if we are literally falling, is easily dismissed by most of us as an illusion carried over from the dream, and the separation between real and imagined is soon re-established.

We might think of this as the 'conventional' modern view of sleep and dreaming, for which a number of assumptions are made:
• Dreams are chaotic and beyond our control.
• The content of the dream is generated by the activity of the brain.
• It is generated solely from within that person.
• The body remains in more or less the same place throughout sleep.

But not everybody takes such a rational view of sleep and dreaming. The falling off tall buildings or dropping at great speed with a sudden jolting of the body is typical of an abrupt transition between sleep and wake. Not so long ago it would be quite normal to decide on an alternative explanation, perhaps that the soul or spirit is caught short by a forced awakening and is hurriedly returning to the safety of the body before full consciousness has returned.

In this chapter, views of the dream as a bridge between rational and non-rational experience are explored, along with new prospects in the way we dream: the 'lucid dream'.

'Normal' dreaming

Following the discovery of REM sleep as a discrete state and its coincidence with dreaming, considerable effort went into describing the dream in objective terms. For example, we know that dreams rely on sensory information in just about the same proportions as our waking experience. Practically all dreams have some sort of visual content. Auditory information, usually as dialogue between dream characters or whispers from some 'off-screen' character, follows a close second and is a feature of approximately 70 per cent of all dreams. Touch, taste and smell are far less evident, but when present often represent a more sinister twist. We dream in colour, and we have depth perception, although visual distortions, fuzziness around the edges, blurred vision and fish-eye views are also common. We dream in something close to 'real time'; convoluted and drawn-out dream stories actually take up longer periods of REM sleep than short, snappy dreams. In fact, apart from the bizarre nature of the dream, shifts in time, unpredictability and so on, we could easily be fooled into thinking of a dream as reality.

During REM sleep, although the EEG is active, muscle control is low, so that most of the body (with the obvious exceptions of involuntary functions necessary to remain alive, and the eyes) is effectively paralysed. Normally we are never aware of this, despite frequent shifts into this state throughout the night. This is because of its precise coincidence with sleep and not waking brain states. However, from time to time the mechanisms initiating dream imagery and body paralysis do not work smoothly and in synchrony with each other, resulting in extremely bizarre and often terrifying and perplexing experiences (see Chapter 14).

Dreaming also occurs in other stages of sleep, although this is generally assumed to be qualitatively different to the REM dreaming experience. Two periods of sleep have attracted considerable attention, because of the types of imagery associated with them and the confusion or overlap between the sleep and wake states. The first occurs in the minutes following the initiation of sleep and is described as 'hypnagogic' imagery; the second, 'hypnopompic' imagery, occurs in the confusion of waking (see Chapter 3). With hypnagogic and hypnopompic imagery there is usually an overwhelming sense of being awake, but the mind seems just to drift into a sudden and unexpected intrusion from the imagination. Most people have some experience of these two states, and think nothing of it.

We are also known to dream in NREM sleep, particularly Stages 2, 3, and 4. These types of dreams are more difficult to remember, and tend not to be as bizarre or fantastic as the REM-associated dream. Deep sleep is also linked with other behaviours, especially sleep-walking (see Chapter 14).

Nightmares

The occasional nightmare has to be expected from time to time and is a perfectly normal feature of sleep, although frequent nightmares, particularly with a shared theme, can point to some underlying psychological difficulty. The most terrifying nightmares are thought to begin in the deeper stages of NREM sleep. These are quite different to the narrative-type REM dreams.

Nightmares from Stage 3 and 4 NREM sleep tend to focus on a particularly terrifying theme, often centred around death or violence. Waking is abrupt, sometimes with shouting or screaming. The heart is racing and confusion or terror persists for several minutes. These nightmares, often referred to as 'night terrors' to distinguish them from the REM nightmare, usually occur in the first half of the night, when the deeper stages of NREM sleep are more prevalent.

It is not uncommon during this type of nightmare to be attacked or chased by visiting monsters, especially small demon-like creatures (incubus and sucubus), savage animals, vampires, werewolves or other blood-sucking or life-threatening forces. Early psychodynamic theory interpreted these dream characters as veiled references to forbidden, often incestuous, desires. The consequence of such a taboo desire is played out in a nightmare, in which the forbidden sexual partner (typically a parent or close family friend) is represented as a devouring monster. Thus the overwhelming fear stems from the fear of punishment and an awareness of moral condemnation. In this view, the nightmare can remind us of the moral and social boundaries governing acceptable and non-acceptable behaviours.

The nightmare can also be a repetition of an actual experience. Although usually transformed, the scenario of a distressing experience is replayed, thus providing a sometimes therapeutic opportunity to come to terms with the event. When this happens shortly after a major trauma, the connection is obvious. But the nightmare can sometimes mask experience for which an actual memory is repressed and long forgotten.

Nightmares have also been linked with actual bodily sensations, particularly poor digestion (related to milk products), circulation or precocious sexual arousal in children. Creatures which are especially tickly and crawly, such as spiders and crabs, are regular visitors in this category and have been thought to be the imaginary representation of actual bodily sensations.

Extraordinary dreams

Physiological, psychological and cultural interpretations

A surprisingly large number of people claim to experience extraordinary dreams, whose properties – visits from non-humans, separation of the body and soul, astral travelling – often defy rational, scientific explanation. There are often huge differences in the ways these events are interpreted. From the individual's point of view, many of these events are terrifying, distressing or difficult to understand, while others are able to see them in a positive light and explore them with obvious enjoyment. From a scientific point of view, it does not make sense to ignore the scale of these experiences. While the interpretation is often questionable, the subjective experience is nevertheless valid. Just as with the precognitive dream, the fact that so many people describe these experiences and believe them to be real (surveys often find that any-thing up to seven out of ten people accept this possibility) suggests that we should not be quick to dismiss or trivialize them. These are real experiences – they impact on people's lives, influencing their behaviours and beliefs.

Out-of-body experiences

Estimates suggest that a substantial proportion of the population of western societies currently believe in the possibility of an 'out-of-body' experience. At its simplest, 'out-of-body' refers to a sense of separation between the physical matter of the body and the mental experience, whether that is the mind, the soul, the spirit, the astral body or whatever. Accounts of these experiences vary enormously, yet their prevalence during sleep suggests that this is a time of particular vulnerability or sensitivity to these events. There is extensive anecdotal evidence for this concept throughout history, as it has been invested with considerable cultural significance over the years. But what could the significance possibly be nowadays, for a modern world whose mainstream scientific position is sceptical of such things being anything other than perceptual distortions?

There are many reasonable explanations in terms of physiological or psychological factors to account for dissociation between the body and mental activity. During sleep most of us are content to submit to a loss of body awareness and remain assured that the body exists. Even during dreaming, when the mind is extremely active, we are not preoccupied with the body or our memory of it. When we go to sleep at night we expect to remain, both body and soul, intact and within the confines of our bedroom – or do we?

In the USA in the early 1980s, over 1,500 people responded to a national newspaper article about 'out-of-body' experiences, in which readers were invited to send in detailed accounts of their own experiences[1]. A sample was then selected at random and these people were sent questionnaires about the circumstances and details of their out-of-body experiences, and how they themselves made sense of them. They were also asked to provide more general information about religious and spiritual beliefs, events dominating their lives at the time of the experience, and how their outlook or beliefs about such things had been changed, if at all.

One of the most significant findings from this study was that there was no such thing as an average 'believer'. Instead, the respondents came from a wide background in terms of age, economic status, occupation and lifestyle, thereby ruling out any obvious stereotyping that the idea of out-of-body experiences might attract. Both men and women responded, (about the same number of each), some married and some single.

As with precognitive dreams, over half the respondents reported having had an out-of-body experience more than once, suggesting perhaps that they had a certain sensitivity towards these experiences. Alternatively, it may be that they were more willing to admit to them and go to the effort of responding to a newspaper article. Over one-third had their out-of-body experience during dreaming but were adamant that this was not a simple dream experience. Although it is often assumed that the out-of-body experience is triggered by a near-death episode (eg during surgery), this was not a strong finding. More general assumptions concerning psychological vulnerability were also unfounded, with less than one-quarter of this group reporting to be in a heightened state of emotional distress immediately prior their experience. The questionnaire also revealed that almost one-quarter were actively involved with or believers in psychical possibilities, and that around 10 per cent of all out-of-body experiences reported were believed to be induced rather than completely spontaneous. Techniques for inducing or perpetuating out-of-body experiences are now widely available, and often cover a spiritual dimension.

So what is the out-of-body experience like? Descriptions vary from the vague feeling of being loose or separate from the body, to actually visualizing the body from an onlooker's position. Almost all accounts agree that the experience is 'more real than a dream' – although the dream may be necessary at the outset to facilitate the experience. In the American study, very few of the respondents felt that their out-of-body form had changed in any significant way from their physical form, and just over half remained close to their physical body throughout. Many of them also described the experience as 'energizing' and saw it as a positive or non-threatening experience. Bright light and the presence of a friendly force featured in a small number of cases, but perhaps not as much as we might assume, given the nature of the more well publicized forms of out-of-body events.

On the whole, this was not a frightening experience and the overall effects were generally comforting. What is clear is that the out-of-body experience is seen as a meaningful one – the effects of which, in terms of emotional well-being or spiritual calm, can be long lasting. Finally, as this survey was purely voluntary we have no real idea how many people share similar experiences but prefer to rationalize them in more logical terms.

Cross-cultural studies[2] have found that the out-of-body experience is not only widespread throughout the world (about 95 per cent of the cultures studied), but also that there are many similarities between the descriptions despite vast differences in terms of cultural complexity, religious base and geographical location.

Sleep paralysis

Alien abductions are on the increase, or so it seems. Science has offered a rather simple and perhaps mundane account of these claims, yet many staunch believers in the UFO phenomenon remain unconvinced. Stories of physical interference or even abductions during sleep by alien or ungodly forces describe how the victim is completely paralysed during an attack, yet wide awake and fully aware of events as they unfold. It has been pointed out that these descriptions are remarkable similar to some aspects of folklore, such as the traditional stories of Old Hag attacks from Newfoundland, and the vampire and werewolf attacks of Eastern Europe.

One simple explanation suggests that this is a form of sleep paralysis, in conjunction with hypnagogic or hypnopompic hallucinations. Sleep paralysis is a normal part of every night's sleep, although waking up to find that we are still partially or completely paralysed is not. Eventually during these 'attacks', the body will regain full consciousness and movement is regained. At its most extreme, however, sleep paralysis can be extremely unnerving: not only is the person unable to move, but they are often also aware of some threatening force in or around the room with them. There is a common thread running through many accounts, involving some or all of the following features:

• Sense of a malevolent of threatening force.
• Shapes in the dark; black or grey shadowy figures near the bed or approaching it.
• Footsteps, breathing, scratching and rasping noises.
• Heavy weight on the chest, leading to a sense of suffocation or choking.
• Complete or partial paralysis.
• Inability to scream or cry out.
• Pain in limbs.
• Unnatural calm.
• Unpleasant smells.
• Overwhelming fear or dread.
• Bodily sensations as if being touched.
• Buzzing sensation in the ears or other auditory distortions.

Depending on which survey you rely on, anything up to 40 per cent of the population are thought to experience sleep paralysis in some form or another, either frequently or as a one-off experience. The episode can last from a few seconds to many minutes – although time estimation in this highly aroused state is questionable.

So what is happening? Monsters and demons have always, sensibly, favoured the sleeping victim. From the incubi and sucubi (demons with sexual predilections) of medieval times to the modern alien, sleep offers a unique opportunity for evil intent. By first paralysing the victim, the attacker is free to do as they wish. But sleep is also a difficult state to assess subjectively. How far does the hallucination explanation account for these attacks?

Arousal from REM sleep

The transition between sleep and wake relies on brain activity and motor control coming into line at the same time. While the EEG of REM sleep is similar to wake, we are normally spared conscious awareness of the motor inhibition leading to paralysis during this state of sleep. This transition does not always occur smoothly, however, and there may be a period of overlap, when there is subjective awareness indicative of wake but the body is still in a state more typical of sleep. Fortunately, this does not occur very often.

The powerful visual and auditory elements of this experience may be some sort of carry-over from the dreaming state. It seems as if there is a delay in the body and elements of mental activity coming into line with full arousal. Sleep paralysis is nearly always associated with unpleasant imagery, suggesting a strong psychological element. For example, most people assume quite early on that the threat is non-human. But it also seems to be relatively benign, sufferers rarely coming to any harm from their experience. Psychologically, the effects can be more long lasting, depending on how the event is understood, either as a physiological anomaly of sleep or as a genuine predatory attack. What is interesting, though, is the vividness of the encounter, which adds to the sense of it being real as opposed to merely a dream. Unlike typical dreams, there is a level of body awareness that we do not usually expect.

Visual and auditory hallucinations are readily described in terms of brain function. However, many accounts of sleep paralysis describe the sensation of being watched or observed without actually seeing or hearing anything. Is this simply another form of sensory distortion? Is it possible that in this state we are hypersensitive to the environment, perhaps at a subconscious level? A foreboding sense of danger before an event can sometimes be triggered by subtle changes in the environment which we do not consciously register (as with certain dreams which appear to be precognitive – see Chapter 10). It seems that when we are awake we have an almost uncanny ability to sense when we are being stared at, even though we may be facing in a completely different direction. If there is any truth in this, then it would not be unreasonable to expect further distortions during sleep, especially during a state of confusing sensory input.

A similar sensory distortion might account for the lack of bodily feedback during out-of-body experiences, leading to the sensation of floating without the physical 'anchoring' of the body. In this sense, a much tamer description would be to say that we are out of touch with the body, rather than outside the body.

Coping with sleep paralysis

At one time, sleep paralysis was considered to be part of the narcoleptic syndrome (see Chapters 3 and 12), because of the similarity in perceptual disturbance around the onset of a narcoleptic attack. It is now recognized that attacks of sleep paralysis also occur independent of other symptoms of narcolepsy, particularly the rapid, overwhelming urge to sleep during the day.

Most of these episodes end spontaneously, although this may be little comfort at the time. For some people, waking up to temporary paralysis can be a fairly regular experience – so much so that they devise their own 'strategies' to bring about an early termination or transform the situation into a less negative experience. For example, as paralysis is rarely complete, concentrating effort into moving a finger or a toe can often be enough to break through and restore full movement.

Acute sleep deprivation is know to be a factor in increasing the chances of a sleep paralysis episode, and should be avoided by maintaining a regular schedule of sleep and minimizing stress and anxiety as far as possible. Relaxation techniques before sleeping can help. For some reason, lying on the back, rather than on the side or face down, seems to be a trigger, and is five times more likely to be associated with an attack than other positions. Regular sufferers also advise relaxing during the paralysis rather than fighting it, concentrating on positive imagery or thoughts as far as possible. Many have learned to transform the paralysis attack into a more benign episode, such as the out-of-body experience, in which they have relatively more control. Struggling doesn't seem to help, and anecdotal accounts describe this as 'feeding' the terror.

The long-term impact of these experiences really depends on how they are understood. Very often, it is the vividness of the event which distinguishes it from a normal dream and persuades the individual that something extraordinary is happening. Combined with the overwhelming sense of threat or danger, there has always been a tendency to rely on non-human sources, in one form or another, to explain these events. It has been suggested that the alien abduction theory is simply the current way of understanding an age-old phenomenon, with the religious or demonic spectres replaced by a more up-to-date threat: the technologically advanced extra-terrestrial.

In many ways, this account of sleep paralysis does give a reasonable and rational explanation of what might be happening during 'abduction' episodes, and people who are willing to accept this tell similar stories to those who opt for the alien interpretation. When the information coming from the body and the senses is unusual and confusing for us, it is not surprising that we should look for an explanation beyond our normal understanding. However, this does not explain why some people are more vulnerable to these attacks than others.

Other explanations

It has also been suggested that perhaps many experiences believed to be paranormal are simply by-products of the brain, specifically the temporal lobe areas. Among their many functions, the temporal lobes handle information from the sense organs (sight, sound, taste, smell, touch), in addition to body positioning and awareness. Patients whose brains are stimulated in this area during brain surgery under local anaesthetic have been known to report out-of-body experiences, a sense of a presence and other extraordinary events. So, in the case of sleep paralysis, for example, perhaps everything is a powerful hallucination, right down to the sense of dread, buzzing in the ears, sulphurous smell, cold chill in the room and dislocation from the body?

Brain wave patterns – particularly the idea of alpha activity – are also thought to be conducive to paranormal experience. During alpha activity, the brain is in a state of peaceful vigilance and relatively free from distraction or engagement. This is not quite so sleepy as theta activity, or as active as beta waves. Consequently, people focus on the alpha 'rhythm' for inducing alternative, trance-like states of consciousness.

Paranormal experiences have also been linked with melatonin output, a substance which is produced predominantly during the night-time period, and geophysical activity. In the latter case, this often involves linking retrospective reports of geomagnetic or seismic activity with the reporting incidence for paranormal events. None of these approaches questions the truth of claims of paranormal activity such as premonition, telepathy or alien visitors – they are more concerned with coincidences surrounding the timing of such reports. Although the underlying mechanisms to explain any association remain unclear, the suggestions seem to be that environmental conditions somehow impact on the activity of the brain to produce these experiences.

Finally, perhaps we cannot expect such a limited view of the dream as the one described at the start of this chapter. Rather than thinking of sleep and wake as two separate states, it seems that there are periods when there is sufficient overlap between the two to produce bizarre, transient states. Although not all of them are welcome, some are positively enjoyable.

Lucid dreams

Lately, there has been enormous enthusiasm for the idea of lucidity during dreaming. Although this concept has been around for many years, for some reason it has only recently captured the public's imagination. It is nevertheless taking off in a big way and promises to open up a new dimension of experience for the average, not just the gifted, dreamer.

Normally we would only expect to know about a dream when we wake up, if at all. Recall of dreams is also notoriously unpredictable, and many people will claim that they never dream, even though their EEG and other objective indications suggest otherwise. And yet it seems that there are ways of taking a more active role in this process.

Dream 'lucidity' refers to the idea of having awareness and control during an actual dream. The attraction lies with crucial differences between the lucid and non-lucid dream: non-lucid dreams are identified only in retrospect, not as they happen, and there is no volition or control – we are nothing more than passive voyeurs. In contrast, the lucid dreamer is limited only by the scope of their imagination. During lucid dreaming, a person:

• Is aware of being in a dream as it happens.
• Controls the flow of the dream.
• Determines who is involved.
• Can think clearly about the experience as it happens.
• Can make deliberate actions and reflect on them.
• Can remember the circumstances of normal waking life (family, home, friends, work, etc).

So who can have lucid dreams? Everybody, apparently. There are now many devices on the market to assist in recognizing the onset of a dream. Most of these rely on some sort of external monitoring device, targeting eye movements, respiration or muscle tone, for example. When these devices pick up evidence of a shift into what is presumed to be REM sleep, then a signal is sent to the sleeper to alert them to this fact (this should be sufficient only to rouse them gently rather than wake them). The idea is that by learning to recognize the dream state, one is half-way to taking a more active role in its outcome. Sceptics have argued that these devices simply arouse the sleeper to a level of confused drowsiness, and so effect something like a 'day-dream', ie a waking fantasy.

But the evidence for some awareness during dreaming is really quite strong. In controlled studies, for example, experienced lucid dreamers are able to signal to an observer when a dream starts. These signals, usually in the form of a pre-discussed eye movement, generally correspond well with objective measures, such as the EEG, to confirm that the person is asleep and not simply drowsy. It seems that some people really do know when they are dreaming, and are sufficiently lucid to remember the arrangements of their waking reality in order to communicate this awareness to the outside world. For advocates of the lucid dream, this represents clear evidence that it is not simply a confused state bordering on wake.

So what are the benefits of lucid dreaming? It is claimed that there are many, from simply having more fun to gaining more insight into the dreaming process and the world of the inner self. Business, social and sporting skills can all be practised and honed to perfection during the lucid dream state. The lucid dreamer controls location, characters and plot. Flying is recommended, as is any activity you would not normally expect to get the chance to take part in during wakefulness. However, the lucid dream is not to be confused with the out-of-body experience as, by definition, the lucid dreamer knows that an activity is not real, whereas with the out-of-body experience this is not always clear at the time.

What are the drawbacks? According to the promoters of the lucid dream, there are none, whereas followers of the psychodynamic approach are more sceptical. In keeping with Freud's original theories, the dream is supposed to be unpredictable, difficult to understand and soon forgotten. The principal function of dream time is to resolve our innermost secret conflicts, which are too sensitive to be brought into conscious awareness. If we block this process by introducing lucidity into our dreams, then when can this function – which is believed to be essential for emotional well-being – be achieved? Proponents of lucid dreaming have also attracted criticism for even wanting to control an experience that is best left in its chaotic and disorganized 'natural' state.

Where now?

So, where are we when we sleep? It seems that the possibilities are expanding all the time. By exploring the potential of different states or levels of consciousness, the lucid dream empowers the individual, while also helping to shed light on unusual dream or sleep states which we normally consider to be non-voluntary – such as the paralysis attack or the spontaneous out-of-body experience.

For many, the ability to recognize dreams as they happen and influence their outcome is first realized as a strategy for dealing with unpleasant sleep experiences, such as sleep paralysis or nightmares. Further down the line, there may be a problem here which has relevance to the cases of sleep-related physical behaviours discussed in Chapter 14. At the moment, sleep is understood in many legal contexts to be a state of mind lacking volition or intent, and there are many cases involving sleep-related behaviours which have relied on this fact. If we all become expert lucid dreamers, does this mean we also take on the responsibility for behaving ourselves during sleep?

Despite early enthusiasm for the dream, the functions of dreaming remain unclear. Dreaming is rarely problematic and this is perhaps why it is not quite so high on the scientific agenda as many would like. Accepting the diverse range of dream experiences may allow people to be more comfortable with what is happening to them and perhaps take a more positive view. In many ways, though, today we have trivialized dreams to the point where for many people it would be uncomfortable to be seen to be taking their dreams too seriously.

Part 4

Sleep in a modern world

Chapter 12
What's left to explore?

We are told that we spend almost one-third of our life asleep, and yet the essential reasons for this remain unclear. At least 100 years of scientific endeavour in laboratories around the world have been dedicated to sleep and, despite many advances, the questions continue to accumulate. In the last 20 years alone there has been enormous interest in this area, with hundreds of research programmes geared towards understanding not only the basic physiological reasons for sleep, but important social and environmental issues raised as a consequence of living in a more complex and demanding society. From the early and perhaps extreme experiments of the 1900s to today's emphasis on getting to grips with the idea of a 24-hour society, a huge industry of sleep-related clinical and research programmes has emerged, all engaged at some level in this fascinating area.

Modern sleep research has highlighted the importance of dealing with a wide range of sleep disorders suffered by significant sections of the population. Narcolepsy, virtually unheard of in the early part of this century, is now familiar to many. Sleep apnoea is discussed regularly on news, health and magazine programmes, suggesting increased public awareness for a debilitating illness thought to affect approximately two per cent of the population to some degree.

In the workplace, sleep research has contributed substantial pragmatic expertise in dealing with the problems of shiftwork, from scheduling and rotating of work schedules to workstation design. In the home, research has contributed to a greater understanding of the problems of insomnia, including social and environmental issues which are often important factors in the emergence of sleep difficulties. Recent research into dreaming has provided the opportunity to explore the idea of subconscious motivations, in addition to offering alternatives to the conventional dream state.

The aim of this chapter is to explore the issues on today's agenda, given the continuing public and scientific interest in this topic. Ongoing research can be categorized broadly into the following areas:
• Sleep medicine.
• Sleep, the body and the brain.
• Behaviours during sleep.

• Behaviours during sleep loss.
• Sleep and work.
• Sleep and ageing.
• Dreaming.

However, it is rarely this clear cut, with many areas providing overlap between related issues. For example, research into sleep loss, work-related issues and sleep medicine all contribute towards the more general questions of how much sleep we need, and why.

Sleep medicine

Disorders of the mechanisms controlling peaceful, restorative sleep at a time convenient to our daily lives are currently the focus of much scientific and medical interest. Although there is nothing new about such disorders, it is only recently that scientists have begun to understand their prevalence in society and have responded to a pressing need for more effective treatment strategies.

By increasing awareness of sleep disorders, this drive has allowed people to come forward with symptoms which had previously been suffered either as part of the normal ageing process or simply dismissed as characteristic of that individual.

Narcolepsy

Narcolepsy is a disorder in which sufferers experience the sudden and over-whelming urge to sleep. The need to sleep is extremely powerful and difficult to avoid, and can occur at anytime of the day and under many otherwise stimulating and perhaps dangerous circumstances.

A narcoleptic 'attack' is often found in association with cataplexy (loss of muscle tone), in which the individual is effectively unable to control their body and may drop abruptly to the floor. Emotional arousal such as laughing, crying or other forms of excitement can trigger such an episode. It is also common to have unusual, perhaps bizarre imagery around falling to sleep.

Treatment for narcolepsy is typically targeted towards the regulation of sleep in order to avoid such attacks during the day – stimulants such as amphetamines may be prescribed to maintain alertness during the day and enhance sleep at night. Sufferers (narcoleptics) generally get a normal amount of sleep, although both the timing and level of urgency are abnormal. It has been known for some time that narcolepsy runs in families, not only with humans but also with other animals, including dogs. It is thought that there are currently around 10,000 diagnosed narcoleptics in the UK alone.

Although there are other explanations for being excessively sleepy during the day, narcolepsy can be distinguished from these because of the unusual timing of sleep 'attacks'. This is especially true if they occur when we would expect almost nil circadian-related pressure, nil social pressure, and nil 'build-up' of a need for sleep, ie time from last sleep. The daytime 'naps' in themselves, although short, can be refreshing. Narcoleptics also show a characteristic REM period shortly after sleep onset (whereas for most people this is normally delayed until sleep is more firmly established), a factor which again helps with clinical confirmation.

Although narcolepsy has been recognized for many years, recent research has been able to offer a clearer picture of the underlying physiological mechanisms and genetic features responsible for this disorder. However, so far treatment has focused on management of the main symptoms rather than a cure. For the narcoleptic, the added indignity of disbelief or even ridicule at the idea of falling asleep without control in public places must be endured.

Sleep apnoea

Estimates suggest that approximately five per cent of men and three per cent of women suffer from some form of sleep apnoea, although there are suspicions that even higher levels go undetected.

Sleep apnoea is a condition of disordered breathing during sleep, in which breathing stops for a short period and until such time as the person gasps for breath, usually with sufficient effort to awaken momentarily. This can happen many times during the night, and although these short awakenings may not be remembered, the consequences of continuous disturbance during the night can have devastating effects the next day, leading to an overwhelming sense of sleepiness and lack of energy, and an increased risk of falling asleep unexpectedly. For that reason, a number of countries do not allow individuals diagnosed with sleep apnoea to drive without evidence of successful treatment over a sustained period.

Two broad categories of sleep apnoea have been identified: obstructive sleep apnoea (OSA) and central sleep apnoea. OSA is the more common form, with a higher incidence among middle-aged obese men than other groups. In OSA, a narrowing of the airway blocking or restricting air flow impairs breathing. After a short period (ranging from a few seconds to more than a minute), a rapid gulping of air restores the airway. This leads to a brief awakening from sleep which may not last long enough to be remembered, but repeated hundreds of times is sufficiently disturbing to have a serious impact on the restorative value of sleep.

The more obvious symptoms include heavy snoring (more likely to be noticed by a partner than the person actually snoring), unsatisfying sleep, and overwhelming sleepiness during the day. In addition, sleep apnoea can also have less direct or obvious effects on work performance and social relations – for example, it can be extremely difficult for a partner to live with. There is a range of treatments currently available for OSA, usually designed towards restoring air flow, including surgery to remove excess tissue or devices worn over the nose designed to keep the airway open by literally blowing in pressurized air.

With CSA, there is no obvious airway obstruction and the source of the problem is considered to lie within the brain. During sleep, the signal to breathe is either weakened or lost momentarily, and the sufferer relies on a more voluntary or 'behavioural' drive to breathe established during wake. Central sleep apnoea is less common than OSA, or may also occur in combination with some degree of OSA.

Both forms of apnoea interfere with sleep, hence the ongoing problems with sleepiness during the day. Because of the frequent disruptions during sleep, time spent in the essential, deeper stages of sleep is dramatically reduced. Sleep apnoea is nowadays considered to be one of the main targets deserving of further research because of the serious impact of it on quality of life, and recent statistics to show that sufferers of sleep apnoea are a particularly high-risk group for accidents because they suffer from excessive sleepiness during the day.

Insomnia

Insomnia has become one of the major torments of the modern age, for which the distractions of a busy lifestyle and erratic, often demanding activity schedules are held to be responsible.

Literally meaning 'to be without sleep', insomnia is used in everyday language to describe all extremes – from the odd night on which it takes just a few minutes longer than usual to fall asleep, to years on end of predictable nightly frustration and the sense of sleeping for just minutes rather than hours. It is often the *perception* of not having had enough sleep, as well as quantifiably poor sleep, which must be taken into account when assessing the severity of an insomniac's complaint.

Although in the normal sense insomnia covers many unique circumstances, a few distinctions as to the cause and possible treatment approaches can be made:

• *Breakdown of physiological mechanisms controlling sleep onset and sleep continuity*. This is unusually difficult to establish, because of the ongoing influence of social and environmental factors in determining how well and when we sleep. It is also relatively difficult to break out of a cycle of reinforcement for sleep problems which, although physiological at source, are exacerbated further by the constant disappointment and frustration of not being able to sleep, thus establishing powerful psychological barriers to sleep in addition to the original problem.

'Physiological' insomnia may be treated with long-term drug use and/or behavioural sleep 'hygiene' regulation to schedule sleep attempts during times most favourable to a successful outcome.

• *Underlying difficulties – social, psychological and environmental.* Whether they be financial, work- or family-related problems, for some people it is as if as soon as their heads hit the pillow the worst of their daily worries jump to the forefront of their mind and refuse to budge. Although we can predict difficulties around many life events, such as a house move, new baby, loss of partner, etc, sometimes there will be no obvious reason other than feeling generally unsettled or anxious. Sleeping pills can help in very stressful situations, but it is more important to get to the root of the problem if good quality, natural sleep is to be restored.

• *Long-term sleep problems.* These often develop as a result of anxiety about sleep long after the initial problems have been resolved. Relaxation techniques (physical and mental) in combination with sleep 'hygiene' can help to some extent, by the sufferer learning to avoid intrusive thoughts which interfere with the process of falling asleep. It is also important to develop a more positive association with sleep: going to bed anxious and concerned about the idea of another restless night is self-fulfilling. Alcohol and an over-reliance on sleeping pills should be avoided as far as possible, as it is important to feel in control rather than dependent on some artificial means of falling asleep.

Advice along these lines often encourages insomniacs to be less concerned with the amount of sleep they think they need each night, and more positive about actual sleep gained. It is tempting for people who have difficulty sleeping at night to take sleep whenever they can get it, and some may resort to napping during the day. In these circumstances, it is very likely that daytime sleep will only add to the difficulties experienced at night, and the importance of maintaining a regular and disciplined schedule of sleep is stressed.

• *Illness.* As pain and health concerns often interfere with sleep, particularly at night, there is now considerable interest in the treatment of insomnia as a symptom of unrelated physical illness.

• *Substance abuse.* We often interfere with the natural process of sleep, perhaps without realizing, through the excessive use of caffeine, alcohol, etc. This can be avoided easily by either cutting down or cutting out consumption of such substances at around the time we would normally expect to be winding down for sleep. And yet we seem to be consuming more caffeine than ever before, prompting suggestions that we are in fact propping an already flagging system as an alternative to facing up to the fact that we are tired and ready for bed. Despite subjecting the system to an ongoing diet of alerting substances, we expect an almost instant reaction when we are ready to sleep.

• *Not knowing we are asleep.* For a small proportion of insomniacs, the difficulty lies with being able to know when they are actually asleep. We normally expect to have a memory of being asleep after just one or two minutes of light sleep, whereas this may actually be much further down the line for some people. Feedback techniques are under development to 'retrain' these individuals so that they are able to recognize sleep when they might previously have felt themselves to still be awake. This approach would obviously benefit from a more thorough understanding of the processes involved in falling asleep, particularly the coincidence between the mechanisms of the procedure (ie changes in the physical state) and the way it is experienced.

• *Novel treatments*. These make frequent additions to a plethora of over-the-counter remedies, the influence of electromagnetic fields generated around the head being one of the latest to emerge.

More and more people are complaining about insomnia, in that they are either genuinely not getting enough sleep or they believe they are not. Either way, it is important to prioritize a good sleep routine, with adequate time set aside for sleep, if the ability to fall asleep easily – something most of us take for granted – is to be preserved throughout adulthood, and despite the vicissitudes of modern life.

Restless leg syndrome

Frequent twitching of the leg muscles is common in later life, but also during pregnancy. This can be extremely irritating and sufferers will often feel dissatisfied with sleep in the morning.

Sleep eating disorder

Details of this disorder have only recently started coming to light. Sufferers binge-eat during the night, usually when they are sleep-walking, and have no recollection of it in the morning. Often the only evidence is an empty refrigerator or signs of food preparation. Women are more likely to eat during sleep than men, although there is no reason to expect the same women to have eating problems during wake. Fortunately, this is quite a rare complaint, but it has potentially serious consequences in terms of weight gain, and risk of injury during cooking or food preparation.

Body clock problems

The importance of the 'body clock' or circadian system and its effects on a wide range of internal processes has been known for some time, although recently this system has been under increasing pressure due to the introduction of many environmental features which are known to interfere with its function. The following conditions are difficult to reconcile with normal, everyday patterns of behaviour, and as such, attract treatments aimed towards bringing the circadian system into line with social expectations.

Delayed sleep phase syndrome (DSPS)

With this condition, the body runs to a 'day' longer than 24 hours and the sufferer feels the need to go to sleep later each successive night. DSPS can be particularly depressing to live with because of the difficulties involved in getting on with a normal working life – sufferers often end up feeling extremely tired when they would prefer to be awake (ie at work or school) but fully alert when they want to be asleep (at night).

There has been some recent success in this area with bright light treatment, particularly when it is timed for early morning, as this approach can help to kick-start the body into action. Light blocks the production of melatonin (associated with increasing sleepiness), thereby offering some relief from early-morning drowsiness. (Light has also been used to speed up adaptation to a different time zone, thereby shortening or reducing the discomfort of jet lag.)

There is a natural shift in sleeping patterns towards DSPS (but not normally to the same extreme) which occurs for many teenagers around the onset of adolescence. Evidence suggests that the sudden and often dramatic shift towards later nights is just as much a biological imperative as it is a social one.

Advanced sleep phase syndrome (ASPS)

With this condition the body runs to a 'day' shorter than 24 hours, so the sufferer feels the need to go to sleep earlier and earlier with each successive night. ASPS is less common than DSPS. Again, treatment with bright light, this time during the evening, can help encourage the body into a more desirable pattern of sleep/wake.

In both the above conditions, the normal 'fine-tuning' of the circadian system to a 24-hour day facilitated by environmental features is inadequate for some reason. Current treatment is aimed towards limiting the discomfort and reducing the social consequences of these conditions.

Sleep related to other physical conditions or illnesses

Sleep problems often emerge in coincidence with the onset of physiological or psychiatric illnesses unrelated to the actual mechanisms of sleep. Huntington's disease, Parkinson's disease, epilepsy, multiple sclerosis, arthritis, rheumatism, migraine, Alzheimer's disease and chronic fatigue syndrome all show a high incidence of sleep-related complaints. Around 60 per cent of all diagnosed cases of depression include complaints about poor quality sleep; this can be both oversleeping – excessive lethargy, lack of energy and drive, etc – and undersleeping – difficulty in getting to sleep, staying asleep or early-morning waking. Abnormal patterns of sleep are also common in other psychiatric conditions, such as schizophrenia and mania. Even the benefits of a short stay in hospital can often be undermined because of the difficulties involved in sleeping in a strange environment, where distractions throughout the night are commonplace. Clearly there is a need to treat sleep difficulties as an important issue in the event of illness, as their effect on overall suffering must not be underestimated.

Sleep, the body and the brain

The technology to produce images of the brain during sleep has provided a unique opportunity to 'snapshot' the brain as the process unfolds, allowing scientists to discriminate between those areas of the brain which seem to have the greatest involvement and those areas which are least active during sleep.

Although promising to unravel many of the ongoing mysteries of normal sleep by providing a new level of description and understanding, this research is in its infancy. It is still both puzzling and infuriating to note that, whether we spend a day on the couch watching rubbish on the television or busily engaged in a more active or intellectually demanding pursuit, the amount we sleep at night is hardly affected. From this, it might seem reasonable to assume that a considerable proportion of sleep is just habit and expendable, so providing further ammunition for the view that people who sleep for long periods are work-shy and self-indulgent.

It is perhaps too obvious, though, to expect a simple trade-off between physical or mental activity expended during wakefulness and hours of sleep needed to restore the body to its previous condition, particularly as the mechanisms for achieving that restoration are still hotly debated. In crisis or self-imposed conditions of sleep loss, such as the impressive marathons of nine to ten days, the body seems remarkably well equipped to do without sleep. Nevertheless, the few studies looking at sleep length and mortality suggest that a normal pattern of eight hours' sleep per night might be a good investment in the long run, although why this should be is unclear. There are also interesting parallels to be drawn from animal sleep patterns, particularly in relation to questions of environment, evolution or security in influencing a drive for sleep.

The study of circadian rhythms also holds much promise for an understanding of the mechanisms involved in the timing of sleep, and provides greater insight into the problems of sleep in the real world. Unusual environments, using either isolated chambers or more natural extreme environments such as the polar regions, have generated many exciting advances in the treatment of circadian-related disorders. This work has highlighted the importance of environmental zeitgebers, particularly natural light and social activity, in stabilizing daily rhythms.

Following from these advances, phototherapy or bright light treatment is currently a popular approach to treating seasonal mood disorders thought to be related to internal rhythms, and many relatively new problems of sleep scheduling such as those due to shiftwork or travelling across times zones.

Optimizing the effectiveness of sleep, even when conditions or timing are not in themselves optimal, is a challenge faced by an increasingly large proportion of the population on a regular basis. This is discussed in more depth in the following chapters in relation to sleep, work and the demands of a modern lifestyle.

'Body clock' research has also thrown up interesting links between sleep and mood, and the existence of distinct circadian 'types' in the population, such as morning 'larks' and night 'owls', who would be well placed to gear their activity towards particular times of the day in order to get the most out of their efforts.

Behaviours during sleep

As with sleep disorders, overt behaviours during sleep have always been around, yet it is only recently that causes and possible treatments have received serious attention. For the most part, sleep-walking and/or talking is considered to be harmless and self-limiting. However, scientists now realize that in extremely rare cases this is not so, and various legal issues concerning responsibility and volition during sleep have emerged. It is only during the last ten years or so that the sleep scientist has been asked to make a contribution to this debate (see also Chapter 14).

Behaviours during sleep loss

The ability to go without sleep for days on end continues to intrigue, and on a popular level it seems that many people are still willing to take part in events which involve long periods without sleep altogether, or with only brief naps at set intervals. Most long-distance walking trials, cinema viewing marathons or even 'talkathons' make extreme demands on staying awake.

However, the problems faced by many occupations in going without sleep are usually compounded by extreme stresses at the time: this is almost definitely the case for many military encounters or response by emergency crew to critical situations. Studies in this area, although ongoing, have brought into context the difficulties faced by individuals in these situations when demands of a higher cognitive nature are made. It seems that the ability to go without sleep physically can be no guarantee of the ability to continue functioning at a high level indefinitely. And yet these ideas are often countered by a more pervasive belief that managing without sleep is all a question of willpower. Situations for which this belief is likely to have serious consequences are discussed in further detail in the following chapters.

Sleep and work

As many industries now choose to provide an around-the-clock service, the problems of trying to stay awake while remaining productive and efficient are firmly in the spotlight. A number of high profile accidents have been related to insufficient sleep, prompting further research into the effects of sleep loss on decisions made under stress.

The introduction of a more flexible workforce has also seen renewed interest in the need to sleep out of synchrony with the body's own needs. Fatigue and sleepiness during the day are not only counterproductive, but present serious risks in many situations. Alternatives to traditional sleep patterns, such as well-timed napping as a short-term solution, provide the focus of much interest in occupational settings.

In contrast, the social problems arising from a change in sleep behaviours on such a scale are often underestimated, or minimized. These problems are often endured in combination with the additional stressors of living in built-up urban environments, bustling with continuous noise and activity. As one of the more successful and popular remedies for coping with the demands of a hectic and demanding lifestyle, physical fitness and exercise is believed to have benefits for all areas of life, including sleep.

Sleep and ageing

The need for sleep is reduced or undergoes natural change with increasing age, although why this should be is still puzzling. The elderly usually complain that their familiar pattern of sleep begins to break down – perhaps they sleep at night but wake up early in the morning. There is often some residual tiredness throughout the day and an urge to sleep in early evening or afternoon. Because this period in life coincides with many social changes in behaviour patterns, it is often difficulty to tease apart these factors from a physiological explanation. These changes can be apparent from middle age onwards and can often take people unawares.

A more pressing need to understand the natural ageing process with regards to sleep has been fuelled by recent population changes, thanks to an improvement in life expectancy. More and more people than ever before can now expect to reach their early eighties and beyond, prompting even further concern for the widespread use of sleeping pills in this age group and the difficulties of coping with chronic pain during the night.

At the other end of the scale, many researchers are active in investigating the conditions for adequate sleep in children. Changes in children's bedroom environments in many modern households are thought to place children at risk of not getting enough sleep, although the evidence in this area is currently sketchy. Should that be the case, the effects of not getting enough sleep are poorly understood and sleep-related problems often go unrecognized against the background of more general behavioural problems. And yet we know that children are not good at recognizing sleepiness in themselves: young children in particular are often, on the surface, bursting with energy and enthusiasm for activity as the time for bed draws near. There is also a pressing need to understand the actual development of sleep patterns in children, particularly around the transition between childhood and adulthood, when sleep patterns undergo their most radical and visible changes.

Sudden infant death syndrome (SIDS) and its relatively high incidence during sleep is an area of particular concern. In the past five years, for example, a simple change in sleep position has had an impressive impact in reducing the incidence of SIDS.

Dreaming

Despite a more pragmatic approach to understanding the problems of sleep, dreams continue to attract considerable research interest. Differences between REM and NREM dreaming may help towards understanding many of the more unusual and perplexing sleep states, such as night terrors and sleep paralysis. Awareness of borderline states, which defy easy sleep and wake distinctions, has prompted more research in this area, and may have repercussions for many traditional beliefs concerning these experiences.

As always, the public demand for dream-related information provides an enthusiastic audience for each new innovation in this area, with advances in lucid dreaming particularly welcomed in recent years. In capturing the public imagination, through training courses, books, devices and so forth, interested parties are invited to explore previously uncharted psychic territory from the relative safety of the lucid dream. Auto-suggestive learning during sleep has also emerged as a popular development, although despite a huge market for these techniques, the scientific evidence for enhanced learning during sleep is not particularly supportive.

This approach taps even further into a willingness to see sleep as some sort of unique channel state through which fundamental elements of the psyche can be reached. It is possible, so it is claimed, to improve memory skills, self-confidence or self-esteem, to get rid of self-destructive habits (such as smoking or alcoholism) and to gain greater insight into the workings of the mind, by playing recorded messages directly into the ears during sleep. These messages guide the subconscious sleeping state to a higher level of knowledge. And yet laboratory studies cast serious doubts on the effectiveness of such techniques: it seems that we forget just about anything we hear from the moment we start to drowse until we are fully alert and awake again. Yes, we do monitor the environment during sleep, but this is a very selective monitoring, and although the ears 'hear', there is no reason to assume that the brain is processing the information presented to them.

Consequently, the assimilation and storage of large amounts of information seems doubtful, as there is no evidence to suggest any form of long-term memory processing during sleep. Even as a subconscious plant, the contents of a tape-recorded message during sleep are only likely to be as effective as waking suggestions. On the other hand, it has been shown consistently that the single most important factor in facilitating learning is internally generated motivation to learn. Quite simply – why miss out on the effort, when it is the consciously driven process that is most likely to pay off?

Finally

The above represents only a selective account of sleep-related topics currently under consideration, although the emphasis on a more problem-driven research strategy, as opposed to simple curiosity, is fairly obvious. It is, perhaps, this willingness to respond to the emergence of a wide variety of sleep-related issues over the years which has led to the ongoing success of and interest in the field of sleep research.

From a cultural perspective, it is clear that sleep continues to fascinate on many levels, although a traditional view of sleep as mysterious and perhaps magical has been replaced by a more hard-line approach. For interest in the paranormal aspects of sleep, such as telepathic visitations and precognitive dreaming, although still given serious thought, you may have to look outside mainstream psychology. Instead, it is much easier to find these ideas rationalized in terms of the individual and social consequences of such beliefs, particularly in a society largely antagonistic to suggestions of the paranormal. In historic and anthropological contexts, however, these discussions make for interesting reading[1].

Sleep and the law

O ver the last ten years or so there has been a growing concern for safety issues in relation to sleep and fatigue, particularly in high-risk occupations such as airline pilots, heavy goods vehicle drivers or industrial plant operators, where the consequences of falling asleep on the job can be catastrophic.

Interest in this area has been fuelled largely through the emergence of compelling evidence to show that accident rates across many occupations mirror the body's 24-hour rhythm of sleepiness and arousal, ie the majority of accidents in 'around-the-clock' operations occur during night shifts. This is not simply a question of physical tiredness, as the same pattern is found for both physically and mentally oriented errors. Instead, these facts suggest a profound vulnerability in the human capacity to cope with certain features of the working environment at a time when the body is normally expecting to sleep. In highly automated work environments, productivity and accident rates all show predictable changes according to the time of day, the night shift creating the greatest problems for human concentration and decision-making skills.

Potential disaster

There are many circumstances in which the consequences of falling asleep are potentially fatal – control of cars, lorries, buses, trains, planes and boats, and highly automated work environments all require continuous and expert attention in order to avoid accidents or errors. Despite many of these activities being extremely boring and repetitive, and requiring concentration in itself just to remain awake, drifting off even for a short period can be extremely serious. Add to that long working hours and insufficient, irregular patterns of sleep and you have what amounts to a recipe for disaster – an accident simply 'waiting' to happen.

Although fatigue has always been recognized as a serious problem in terms of productivity in the workplace, current feeling suggests that many employers and policy-makers seriously underestimate the level of danger faced by an over-tired workforce. While we attribute bad moods, tiredness and general irritability to poor sleep, the full extent of the damage is rarely appreciated. Yet insufficient sleep can play havoc with all areas of life. As we move towards more hectic and increasingly demanding lifestyles, it may be that many of us cannot even remember what it is like to feel wide-awake *all* day. Getting to know just how much sleep we need and when we need it can help towards promoting a sense of well-being on a personal level. On the other hand, we can put off the urge to sleep for as long as possible if we so choose. But what about an obligation to be well rested? Is there such a thing?

In 1988 a representative committee of the Association of Professional Sleep Societies published their views on the dangers of sleep-related accidents in the USA[1]. The report presented a damning insight into the state of the nation's attitudes and behaviours towards sleep. The overall costs of sleepiness-related accidents in terms of lost productivity and personal injury was subsequently estimated at between 43 and 56 billion dollars per year for the USA alone.

Insufficient sleep has been linked with many well known major catastrophes, such as the near meltdown of a nuclear reactor at the Three Mile Island nuclear power plant in 1979, the Challenger space shuttle disaster, the Exxon Valdez oil tanker spill, and the Chernobyl nuclear plant explosion, as well as many lesser known potentially catastrophic near misses. All these incidents involved disastrous decision-making during the night-time hours, when the body is normally demanding sleep. Following the Challenger inquiry, a NASA report found that key workers were acutely deprived of sleep in the crucial hours leading up to take-off[2]. In the Three Mile Island accident, plant operators working in the early hours of the morning (between 4am and 6am) missed vital information. On the Exxon Valdez, the officer in charge fell asleep while on duty. Workers at the Chernobyl power plant misinterpreted crucial information due to fatigue.

Yet media reporting of these disasters focussed on the level of human suffering, damage to the food chain, the environment and the ecology, while issues of sleep, fatigue and the fitness of key workers were given a relatively low profile. Investigations concentrated on technical matters, equipment failure and unforeseeable environmental conditions, and yet when we look at the similarities between such disasters, there are telltale signs of fatigue-related problems. While machinery is not subject to rhythmic fluctuations in performance or efficiency, the timing of many of these disasters points towards the role of human fallibility at a time when we would normally expect to be asleep.

One of the first illustrations of this was provided by a Swedish research group in the 1950s. They compared work efficiency and time of day for a large gas installation plant operating on a 24-hour basis[3]. Once an hour, plant inspectors were required to enter a series of meter readings, referring to production and consumption rates for the plant, into a handwritten ledger.

This task, which involved a small amount of fairly routine mental arithmetic, took place throughout the day and night shifts. At the start of each day, entries for the previous 24 hours would be checked carefully for accuracy and manually re-adjusted if necessary.

When researchers examined the ledgers taken over a 25-year period (by literally holding them up to the light and looking for marks from a rubber eraser or crossings out), they found a clear pattern of increased errors for entries made during the night-time hours compared with morning shifts. A secondary peak also showed up around three o'clock in the afternoon. Before this study, there were only hints of day/night differences in work performance through a small number of studies – telephone operators took longer to answer incoming calls, railway workers made more rule violations – but nothing on such an obvious and long-term scale.

These observations are consistent with our current understanding of human error and fatigue. In healthy adults, there are two powerful and predictable factors which contribute to a feeling of fatigue: how long we have been awake and the time of day. The influence of the first factor becomes evident if we attempt to extend our day beyond what we are normally used to. Common sense and personal experience tells us that, for most people, extending the day beyond 18–20 hours will eventually lead to a profound sleepiness, with sleep imminent despite our best efforts to remain awake.

The second factor concerns the daily fluctuations in the body's drive to sleep. Under normal circumstances, our bodies adjust to the approximate 24-hour norm of industrialized societies. We achieve this synchrony with the help of powerful social cues which dictate when to be active and when to sleep throughout the 24-hour cycle (and will obviously depend to a great extent on age and social grouping). Underlying this socially determined pattern of activity is a robust circadian rhythm which determines our arousal state at any particular point in the 24-hour cycle. This cycle waxes and wanes to produce predictable and measurable fluctuations in our drive to sleep. The effect of this cycle is experienced subjectively as fluctuations in our arousal level, with 'low points' being particularly apparent in the early hours of the morning and to a lesser extent again in the afternoon. This rhythm is extremely dependable and will often be maintained despite short-term changes in our daily activity patterns. Many of the problems of night work, for example, stem from the conflict between the timing of the job and the internal demands for sleep during the night.

Current research

An enormous amount of effort has now been put into understanding why workers are more vulnerable to error during the night and how, if at all, conditions can be improved to minimize error. We have recently seen moves towards an overhaul of working practices for certain occupations, in view of an increasing need to understand and adapt towards the need for regular, good quality sleep, if safety is to be enhanced. One of the biggest obstacles is with current dismissive attitudes towards the need for sleep, in a society determined to 'burn the candle at both ends'.

The current debate centres around two issues: (1) the size of the problem and (2) knowing just what the body is capable of and when it is likely to let us down. At the moment, it seems that the greatest concern is with the following areas:

• Falling asleep at the wheel.
• Making time for sleep: rest breaks and work hours.
• Exceptions: who needs sleep?
• Do we know when we are sleepy?

Falling asleep at the wheel

Conventional wisdom: it's avoidable

Driving on the verge of sleepiness is perhaps one of the biggest issues to have emerged in sleep research over the last ten years. Various estimates around the world put the problem of fatalities and serious injuries due to falling asleep at the wheel on a par with drink-driving. A 1994 report from the National Commission on Sleep Disorders (USA) estimated that driver sleepiness was a contributory factor in a staggering 54 per cent of all vehicle accidents in the USA[4]. Although there are wide variations in reports, due mainly to the way these figures are calculated, the overall impression suggests that the extent of this problem is seriously underestimated.

And yet there is nothing new about driving while sleepy. For example, in 1945 a British judge made the following comments concerning a case in which a driver had fallen asleep as he drove along a quiet road early one morning:

> If a driver allows himself to be overtaken by sleep while driving, he is guilty, at least of the offence of driving without due care and attention… because it is his business to keep awake. If drowsiness overtakes him while driving, he should stop and wait until he becomes fully awake.[5]

The case in question involved a young man by the name of Arthur Butterworth. After working all night at a factory, he drove his car into an oncoming group of American soldiers, injuring many of them. His claim to have fallen asleep without warning just a few miles into his journey was originally accepted by the local magistrates as evidence of loss of control through no fault of his own. Consequently, Butterworth was not held to be accountable for the accident and the case was dismissed. However, when the case went to appeal, the court took an entirely different view of the event, as can be seen from the remarks quoted above.

Having reviewed the evidence, Justice Humphreys explained that in his view falling asleep while driving could not be compared with being overcome by a sudden illness or being attacked by a swarm of bees. These were events that were pretty much unpredictable and beyond the control of the driver. Instead, he decided that before falling asleep the driver 'must have known that drowsiness was overtaking him'.

Clearly, with an obvious statutory requirement to remain attentive while driving, it is helpful to be able to say that there is always forewarning before loss of consciousness. In this case, this assumption was made with relatively little difficulty. But it is an assumption based largely on personal experience, for which there was no scientific support at the time and which is today still open to debate. Consequently, the question of culpability in allowing oneself to be overcome by sleep despite the presumed presence of warning signs remains unresolved.

Justice Humphreys assumed that is was the responsibility of the driver to take heed of these warning signs and to pull off the road until such time as he was fit to drive again. Simple enough in principle – but who, if anyone, is going to judge whether this principle has been applied? Unfortunately, the difficulty lies in being able to quantify precisely and objectively how drowsy an individual might be in the period leading up to an accident. Without being able to establish this with a convincing and reliable degree of accuracy, it is virtually impossible to determine whether a duty to take preventative action has been ignored.

We can, of course, consider the context of the event, as with this case, where the driver had just come off a night shift and would be predicted to be sleepier than a fully rested person. Yet the journey was short, and while many people might, quite sensibly, avoid driving for long distances after a night shift, a few miles would perhaps seem more reasonable.

Drink-driving: a lesson to be learned?

Depending on road conditions, and traffic flow, driving a car can be extremely easy. On a clear run, we can go for miles on end without adjusting the controls. Nor is car driving particularly demanding on cognitive functions; most of the time we rely on automatic, well learned, almost casual responses to other traffic and engage in predictable or easily managed manoeuvres. Concentration and reactions are tested only very infrequently. On familiar journeys, we often lose track of events and can cover miles with absolutely no recollection. With very few decisions to make, comfortable seating arrangements and physically undemanding controls, there is nothing to keep us awake – apart from, of course, the very serious matter of staying alive.

This is the point at which many people feel there is nothing else to discuss. Once a year, they get up in the middle of the night, pack all the kids in the car, and expect to drive hundreds of miles on sheer willpower alone – and all because of an urgency to get to a holiday destination without the frustration of peak-time traffic or the bother of an overnight stop. But is this a reasonable risk to take? Is motivation to stay awake while driving, despite its obvious survival function, relied on too heavily in these and similar circumstances? The statistics suggest that this might be the case, and that public perception of the risks of driving without full alertness is seriously underinformed.

It goes without saying that since 1945 there has been a dramatic increase in the number of cars and commercial vehicles on the roads, travelling at greater speeds and with heavier loads. While, for the most part, we now accept the dangers of driving while under the influence of alcohol, we are clearly less concerned with sleep-related dangers.

However, there are certain similarities in driving behaviour during extreme sleepiness and alcohol intoxication. In both states we are slower to react, show a lack of concentration leading to poor lane positioning, drifting, etc, and demonstrate less concern for other vehicles sharing the road. Actual sleep, even light sleep, means that we are not taking in vital information (about the road, the operation of the car and the presence of other road users) and at worst fail to react to even the most dangerous situations. When a driver falls asleep before a crash there is often no sign of braking or avoidance steering, suggesting that there is absolutely no awareness of the impending impact. Consequently, many of these accidents result in fatalities due to relatively high speed on impact.

In England and Wales, there has been a dramatic reduction in positive alcohol 'breathalyser' testing in the last 25 years; despite more people being tested, over 87 per cent were found to be below legal limits of blood alcohol in 1996, compared with just 36 per cent in 1971. Whatever the reasons, social acceptability of drink-driving has undergone radical change, and guessing the limits of the drink-drive laws is no longer considered macho or 'worth a try'. Instead, drivers of all ages are under increasing moral and social pressure to remain completely sober, and not just under threat of legal sanctions. It may be that until such time as there is a similar shift in thinking towards the acceptability of driving while knowingly short of sleep, concerns for this behaviour will remain unheeded.

Professional drivers: a different level of risk?

We tend to assume that lengthy driving periods present more risks as fatigue increases, but how does this affect actual driving behaviours, and what about people who are expected to drive for long periods on a regular basis as part of their job?

Most of the research into this area has looked at the effect of extended driving periods in driving simulators or under controlled conditions, where the risk to the general public can be minimized. The problem with this approach is that you can't get away from the fact that the driver knows there are no genuine risks of injury. Of the few road-based studies, findings confirm what might be expected: drivers do develop a certain sloppiness in their styles as the hours behind the wheel increase. In one example from the late 1960s a group of volunteers, all non-professional drivers, were asked to take part in a 12-hour driving stint (through town centres and along busy, major roads) throughout the course of a single day[6]. By the end of the day, it was clear that drivers were more willing to initiate dangerous or hazardous overtaking manoeuvres – ie when visibility was poorer or by forcing other drivers to adjust their speed or position to allow them to get past – compared with earlier in the drive. And yet in these conditions the risks were genuine.

What about professional drivers, who spend more time on the roads, particularly at night, when the risk of falling asleep is known to be greatest? Is their risk any greater through sheer exposure? Alternatively, do they have special insight into the problem as a result of extensive experience that allows them to develop successful coping strategies?

Concern for the well-being of commercial drivers stems from work in the USA in the 1970s, which showed that accidents were twice as likely to happen during the second half of a long shift (8–12 hours' driving), and suggesting that fatigue may be an important causal factor. More recently, the Federal Highway Administration Office of Motor Carriers published the findings of the Commercial Motor Vehicle Driver Fatigue and Alertness Study, pointing to an alarming degree of sleep problems in commercial drivers[7]. This study was a joint enterprise between American and Canadian organizations, with the principle aim of achieving an objective assessment of the current regulations regarding work hours in relation to actual practices and driver fatigue. Prompted by concerns over long distances and extensive night driving, this research was the combined effort of many private and public interests from both countries.

The study took place over a seven-year period, during which time drivers were canvassed as to their opinions on current regulations. In addition to this, a more extensive study took place. This involved 'in-cab' observations of a selected sample of 80 drivers while they were going about their normal working arrangements. These observations included, among other things, regular EEG recordings to monitor minute-by-minute fluctuations in alertness, both during the normal working day and for 'off-duty' periods. In this way it was possible to assess alertness during driving, and the amount and quality of sleep taken between long shifts. Concentration, reaction times and visual perception were also tested at regular intervals throughout the working shift.

This is believed to be one of the most extensive studies of its kind, with an estimated cost of over $4 million. Unlike laboratory studies, which rely to a great extent on simulated driving by student volunteers, this study concentrated on professional drivers going about their normal, everyday driving tasks. The main findings were in support of regulatory changes, in view of evidence of widespread driver fatigue for this group.

At the time of the study, the US federal hours of service regulations for commercial motor vehicle drivers allowed drivers up to a ten-hour shift (up to a maximum of 70 hours in any eight-day period), providing this was preceded by at least an eight-hour off-duty period (Title 49, Code of Federal Regulations, part 395). These regulations had been around in essential form since the mid-1930s. One of the aims of the study was to produce recommendations regarding future updates, taking into account the radical changes in the trucking occupation, traffic density, speed, etc over the past few decades. In Canada, the law for commercial drivers allowed for a maximum of 13 hours at one stretch (Commercial Vehicle Drivers Hours of Service Regulations, 1994).

Four normal working schedules came under close scrutiny, as shown in Table 2:

Table 2 **North American long-distance driving schedules.**

1 The ten-hour daytime driving shift (USA)	Drivers follow the same daily driving times between 10am and 8pm approx.
2 The ten-hour 'rotating shift' (USA)	Drivers start at 10am approx. on the first day, then start three hours earlier for each successive day. This shift adheres to the mandatory eight-hour break between ten-hour drives, with about one hour to spare.
3 The 13-hour night-driving shift (Canada)	Drivers follow the same nightly driving times between 11pm and 10am approx.
4 The 13-hour afternoon/evening driving shift (Canada)	Drivers follow the same daily driving times between 1pm and midnight approx.

In addition to the physiological and subjective data, monitoring of driving skills was also extensive, including continuous recording of road positioning relative to lane markers and variations in speed. Drivers were filmed throughout a shift, using a front-on view to study facial expressions, eye rolling, glazing, etc, all of which have been associated with the build-up to falling asleep. Cameras were also positioned to give a 'driver's-eye' view of the traffic and road conditions.

Analyses of the vast quantity of data are still far from complete, although preliminary analysis yielded a number of unexpected results. The main findings to date can be summarized in the list that follows.

• *Time of day*. Drivers were far more likely to experience problems of over-whelming fatigue when they were driving through the night. Critical periods could be found between midnight and 8am. During shifts which extended through the night (Schedule 3 and sometimes Schedule 2), drivers showed more signs of sleepiness in their visual appearance, were increasingly likely to drift between lanes, and made more mistakes on brief psychological tasks (measured during drive breaks).

• *Length of shift*. This was found to be less of a factor than might be expected. The difference in drivers' perceptions of sleepiness and outward appearance during ten-hour and 13-hour shifts was negligible during daytime periods. Although drivers complained of feeling more sleepy towards the end of a shift, this seemed to have no detrimental effect on driving during the day.

• *Build-up of fatigue following multiple shifts*. Drivers tended to complain of being increasingly fatigued as the number of consecutive working days increased.

• *Sleep*. Between shifts the drivers felt that they were short of roughly two hours' sleep per night, compared with their 'preferred' amount of sleep. Taken together, the average amount of sleep gained for all drivers was just over five hours per night. This does seem to be cutting things a bit fine. Drivers following Schedule 3, driving 13 hours through the night (11pm–10am) were worst off, with an average of less than four hours of actual sleep between shifts.

• *Individual tolerance*. Over one-third of all drivers showed absolutely no sign of sleepiness or drowsiness during the study, suggesting that there are large individual differences in the ability to cope with the demands of long-distance driving. There were no clues as to whether those with least difficulty were more experienced in terms of years on the job – is it possible to learn successful strategies to ward off drowsiness? Almost half the drivers in this study pulled off the road and took a short nap, thereby supplementing inadequate sleep on an ad hoc basis. This suggests that these drivers are able to recognize when they are no longer fit to drive.

In sum, it seems likely that regulations to limit driving hours miss the mark – it is the timing of driving and its coincidence with an internally driven sleepiness rhythm, rather than the length of the drive which is more important in eliminating fatigue for these commercial drivers. However, as the report points out, whatever benefit is to be gained from avoiding night driving is likely to be lost on increased traffic density during the day. Perhaps the key to this would be to explore individual differences in tolerance. It is clear from this study that there are some people who cope better working at night, and some who have severe difficulties. Aptitude in this regard may be a useful employment criterion.

The truckers themselves pointed out that the maximum driving hours can, in fact, be the main cause of sleepiness problems. Schedule 2, for example, has been designed to make the most of the obligatory eight-hour rest break. Yet as drivers are asked to bring their start times forward every day, they end up sleeping (or resting) at different times with each new day. It has been suggested that a 14 hours on/10 hours off rule would at least allow for a stable 24-hour pattern. However, the problem of getting through a night shift remains unresolved.

Restrictions due to medical conditions

Driving restrictions for individuals suffering from sleepiness-related disorders are very haphazard at the moment. Sleep apnoea and narcolepsy (see Chapters 3 and 12) are the two conditions most likely to be given specific mention in regulatory guidelines, if at all. Without treatment, both conditions present severe hazards in terms of excessive and, at times, overwhelming sleepiness during the daytime. The main risks are from falling asleep inadvertently while driving a vehicle or operating dangerous machinery. Undiagnosed sleep disorders are thought to account for a substantial proportion of motor vehicle accidents.

In the UK, regulations are quite explicit: persons with narcolepsy or sleep disorders likely to cause excessive sleepiness during the day are permanently excluded from holding a commercial driving licence. Temporary licences (one to three years) to drive private vehicles can be granted after successful treatment, but renewal is subject to successful medical review. A similar pattern is in force for sleep apnoea: licences to drive private vehicles are granted on a 12-monthly renewable basis pending successful treatment.

In Canada, doctors are advised that narcolepsy sufferers need to be symptom-free for at least three months before they can be considered suitable for a driving licence. In Australia, narcoleptics are allowed to drive private but not commercial vehicles after three months without symptoms.

In the USA, interstate travel is governed by federal regulations concerning fitness to drive; only a handful of individual states' regulations make specific reference to sleep disorders. In many cases, there is again a requirement for an arbitrary symptom-free period before a licence can be returned. As in the UK, the rules for commercial vehicles are often stricter than for the use of private vehicles.

But how is risk assessed? Inconsistencies in restrictions can be counter-productive in themselves, as drivers may be reluctant actively to seek out treatment for a problem which is likely to deprive them of their income for a lengthy period. This is particularly unfortunate, as available treatments are generally considered to be effective. Many people have objected to the arbitrary delays between diagnosis and renewal of a driving licence: while some areas are confident after six months 'symptom'-free, others prefer 12 months.

There is only one location –the New England state of Maine, USA – which has so far introduced the idea of an objective test to decide whether a person is fit to drive. Before a licence is returned following diagnosis and treatment of a sleep disorder related to daytime sleepiness, evidence that an individual is not likely to fall asleep quickly under sleep-conducive conditions is obtained using the Multiple Sleep Latency Test. This test is an extremely popular clinical tool; it involves simply asking somebody to lie down in a quiet darkened room and, with the EEG as guidance, measuring how long it takes before they slip into light sleep. The same procedure is repeated at two-hour intervals throughout the day – hence the name Multiple Sleep Latency Test, latency meaning interval or delay. The average time taken to fall asleep throughout the entire day is calculated to give an overall score. At the moment, this is the closest we get to an 'objective' measure of how sleepy a person is. Anybody who falls asleep in less than about five minutes on average during the day, and still shows signs of illness at night, is considered to be at a serious risk from falling asleep and, at least in Maine, is not considered fit to be in control of a vehicle.

But there are drawbacks to this type of testing: it is relatively expensive and time consuming, and requires trained personnel in a medical setting. Although there is considerable interest in developing variations along the lines of a practical and easy-to-use test which might be applied in more occupational settings, nothing suitable is available at present. This enthusiasm for a 'sleepiness' test has prompted suggestions for all commercial drivers to be examined regularly as a condition of employment. Not everybody is happy with this idea, however. The main criticism lies with whether we can really judge the likelihood of somebody falling asleep at the wheel, where there is a strong incentive to remain awake (ie the level of risk), by how fast they fall asleep lying on a bed in a safe, quiet, dark room.

Fit to drive?

Very often, falling asleep at the wheel can only be established with hindsight and when the conditions of an accident point clearly to that possibility. There are wide variations in estimates of sleepiness related accidents, as people are often reluctant to admit to coming close to an accident because of drowsiness or having to fight sleep in order to complete a journey. Hence, accident data is often contradictory because of difficulties in establishing cause, and an under-awareness of the risks. Investigations of fatigue-related factors, time of day, length of time driving and break from normal sleeping patterns tend to be under-reported because, until recently, investigators were simply not expected to consider these issues.

After a crash, it is possible to measure with some precision how much alcohol the driver has in their bloodstream. There is no equivalent test for sleepiness. Often the only indication that sleepiness might be a factor is the driver's recent behaviour. If somebody tells you that they haven't been to bed, or slept at all, for the last two nights, you would presumably feel that they are in an unfit state to drive. Certainly, most reasonable people would agree with you. But what about one night without sleep – how sleepy are we after this? This is not a particularly unusual level of sleep loss nowadays – many people expect to drive home safely after working the night shift. Are they safe? Should they be allowed to drive at all? Without a definite measure of 'alertness', the question of whether we are able or fit to drive in relation to how sleepy we are relies on a combination of factors: what seems reasonable to other people, and how we feel. The law says that if we know ourselves to be sleepy, then we must know we are at risk. Failing to stop at this point is to put other people at risk. But do we always know when we are sleepy?

The longer we go without sleep, the faster we eventually fall to sleep. This is a fairly reliable observation. Is there a point where the pressure for sleep is so urgent that we fall asleep almost instantaneously, without any prior warning? These are the problems faced by legislators. There are obvious moves towards addressing these issues, such as regulatory restrictions for known sleep disorders and the suggestion of compulsory reporting by medics following a new diagnosis. At the moment, however, there are few proposals, other than through raising public awareness, for dealing with the problem of sleepiness through self-neglect.

The warning signs

Many government organizations, local authorities, motoring and other interest groups are starting to think ahead on these issues. Campaign topics tend to focus on:
• Raising awareness of the dangers of driving while sleepy.
• Targeting of high risk groups.
• Modification of driver training programmes to cover advice on sleep and fatigue at the wheel.
• Modifications to crash investigation routines to clarify reporting of sleep-related accidents.
• Introduction of more widespread use of 'rumble strips' as an emergency measure to wake the driver drifting off the road.

Although there is obviously still a long way to go with this research, part of the problem lies with being able to convince the public that this is an important issue. A number of clear findings have emerged, from both professional and non-professional drivers, which may help in assessing the level of risk before embarking on a journey:
• *Time of day*. Both night driving (around 3am to 6am) and mid-afternoon are critical periods for falling asleep at the wheel.
• *Road conditions*. Long, boring roads with no other traffic and uninteresting scenery make staying awake while driving difficult.
• *Chronic and acute sleep loss*. Poor quality sleep due to a medical condition or voluntary sleep deprivation is likely to impact on driving performance.

• *Age.* Young men are particularly at risk. This is more likely to be an exposure issue, as for security and social reasons, young women and older men and women are less likely to be travelling long distances on their own at night.

• *Amount of previous wakefulness.* But note that it is possible (due to time of day) to fall asleep even though you may have been awake for just one to two hours.

• *Length of journey.* Time at the wheel is important, but note (as above) that the time of day factor is often the crucial element, so that even short journeys can be risky.

• *Activity before journey.* This applies especially to long work shifts (see the 1945 case above, where the accident occurred at 9am in the morning following an all-night work shift).

• *Ambience.* Overheated and quiet cars are less likely to stimulate the driver into remaining awake.

• *Alcohol.* The effects of alcohol on driving skills are compounded by sleepiness issues such as time of day.

Do drivers know when they are about to fall asleep? The jury is out on this one. At the moment, the general public decides for themselves when they are awake enough to drive. For this, we may rely too heavily on countermeasures such as caffeine and conversation to prevent us from falling asleep: the passenger is just as likely to be sleepy as the driver. A considerable amount of research is currently underway to look into possible 'in-car' countermeasures. Often this takes a very simple view of the process of falling asleep, which, as discussed in Chapter 8, is rarely an 'all or nothing' process. Physical 'warning signs', such as closing the eyelids or eyes rolling upwards, do coincide with falling asleep for some people, on some occasions – but not always. Mechanical unpredictability on this level would almost definitely never be entertained.

Lethal accidents are probably more to do with momentary loss of consciousness rather than deep sleep. Even as we normally fall asleep, there is a waxing and waning between states, often referred to as 'microsleeps'. The first sign of sleep can last just a few seconds and may not even be noticed by the driver. The first few minutes of sleep tend to be a succession of microsleeps, interspersed with wake. While research into in-car monitoring centres on facial or respiratory cues – particularly lowering of the eyelids, infrequent blinks, staring, eye rolling, etc – all these features, although linked with Stage 1 sleep, may be too far down (or off) the road for the warning device to be of any use.

Making time for sleep: rest breaks and work hours

There is an increasing awareness of the need to understand the conditions for effective and safe working environments. Sleep has been mooted as one of the key factors in this debate. In parallel with this interest, science has been able to deliver a growing understanding of the mechanisms underlying human fallibility related to fatigue. It is now possible to make sensible predictions about how well a person will perform on the basis of their recent sleep 'history'. Whether or not this information is reconciled with the demands of the workplace will depend to a great extent on the willingness of industry, governments and workers to make the right moves.

What is the law regarding sleep and work? In the UK, there has been an emphasis over the past 20 years on the deregulation of working practices in order to maximize the flexibility of the workforce. Yet the European Union has only recently introduced a work hours directive, imposing its own restrictions on the amount of time somebody can reasonably be expected to work. The main thrust of this directive concerns the reform and standardization of health and safety issues in the workplace regarding shift lengths and intervals between shifts. Member states of the EU were given until November 1996 to implement its provisions. At the moment there are vast differences in working practices between countries.

The EU directive covers all maximum work hours, breaks, holidays, weekly rest periods and night working. Specifically, there is to be:
• A minimum 11 consecutive hours off in every 24 hours.
• A mandatory rest break for shifts longer than six hours.
• A minimum 24 hours off for every seven-day period.
• A 48-hour maximum working week (on average*).
• An eight-hour maximum shift in any 24-hour period for night workers (on average*).

However, the conditions marked * refer to average figures over weeks and allow for some degree of flexibility. Working overtime is still possible, although it can no longer be enforced by the employer.

But, in recognizing that many professions rely to a great extent on continuity and flexibility in working practices, a number of exceptions were made:
• Managers and decision-makers.
• Family workers.
• Religious workers.

In addition, some professional groups are offered only limited cover and are still free, for example, to work longer than the eight-hour night shift, but within the more general restriction of a 48-hour week. These professions might generally be considered to demand greater continuity of staff attendance and greater flexibility in responding to fluctuations in demand for services, and include nurses, security personnel, essential services personnel (fuel, postal, emergency services, etc), seasonal work, farming, tourism, etc.

The main impact on night working and shiftwork will be the enforcement of a maximum of eight hours worked in any 24-hour period. This is likely to have a serious impact on companies currently using a 12-hour shift system.

Where night workers experience health problems due to the timing of their work, employers are now expected to accommodate them on an alternative shift schedule where possible. For example, given the support of a sympathetic GP a shift worker could argue against working nights altogether on health grounds. This is a particularly controversial area of the directive, the implementation of which is likely to be problematic. Although most night workers receive additional financial payments in recognition of the difficulties associated with this work, employers are hesitant about giving the option to change to an alternative shift by right.

Employees can also expect a minimum rest period of 11 hours for each 24 hours worked. This would make traditional eight-hour shift changes, currently popular within many industries, no longer tenable.

In the UK, feelings towards these changes were mixed, with many companies expressing concern over the need for a flexible workforce, and one that is able to respond to short-term fluctuations in product demand. Yet research has shown that productivity and accident rates are both negatively affected towards the end of a long shift. Simply being there is no guarantee of working safely or effectively.

Work breaks: no guarantee of sleep

Regulations regarding rest breaks and time off between shifts are based on the assumption that, given sufficient time for sleep, this is exactly what reasonable people will do. Quite recently, an early-morning rush hour train in New Jersey, USA, collided with an oncoming train after the driver (who had been on duty for over 14 hours) failed to stop at a red signal. His shift was broken up by a five-hour rest break, during which time he was expected to sleep on one of the train seats. This type of split-shift working arrangement is not unusual, with the assumption that a four- to five-hour break between lengthy shifts provides sufficient opportunity for restorative sleep implicit in the working arrangements of many organizations. Inadequate sleeping arrangements, and badly timed breaks, means that despite time off many people are in a poor state for getting through the remaining hours on duty.

Exceptions: who needs sleep?

Despite recent measures, there are a number of occupations for which sleep is still considered to be an unnecessary luxury. Doctors are a classic example, and often find themselves working under severe conditions, with allowances for sleep being given a low priority. This is particularly the case for junior or newly qualified hospital doctors, whose job involves regular extended on-call or on-duty shifts. Does it make sense to give special consideration to this group? Despite regular and highly publicized campaigns, there is still a reluctance to place work-hour restrictions on this group.

What are the arguments for long working shifts? Are there any benefits during the first few years of a medical career? Advocates have argued that this 'trial by fire' in hospitals enhances training for a number of reasons. Firstly, it is claimed that only through being around to witness the natural development of a disease or illness, from diagnosis through to treatment and resolution, can a junior doctor get an appreciation for the overall picture. This approach also provides continuity of care, which is thought to be of great comfort to the patient, who is not faced with a series of fresh faces with each new shift. But these arguments do not take into account the likely state of a doctor after being awake for over 24 hours or the quality of the decisions they are asked to make. Traditionalists in medical training point out that the currently estimated 80-hour week of a typical junior hospital doctor is already a great improvement on how long newly qualified doctors could expect to work in the past. But this is a very elitist stance and implies that the medical profession is inured to the critical effects of sleep loss. There is simply no reason to expect these individuals to have special immunity from tiredness.

Late one evening in 1984, a young woman by the name of Libby Zion was taken to the emergency room of a New York hospital. She was feverish and in an extremely agitated state. After being treated initially by the examining doctor for an unspecific 'viral syndrome', within hours her condition had deteriorated; she became confused and more agitated, and was eventually physically restrained. Over the next few hours her temperature increased dramatically. Despite efforts to reduce this, respiratory arrest followed and she died a few hours later.

After discovering that the supervising doctor had worked continuously for over 18 hours prior to her admission, her father questioned the soundness of his judgement, considering the likely effects of severe fatigue. Although no criminal proceedings were ever instigated, the case nevertheless attracted substantial media attention. A grand jury investigation into the case was extremely critical of the hospital's policy towards work hours and supervision of junior medical staff[8]. A report of the Grand Jury investigation was later considered by the Ad Hoc Advisory Committee on Emergency Services, who were to produce their own recommendations for the regulation of work hours for newly qualified doctors. These included proposals to:
• Limit emergency staff to 12-hour shifts.
• Limit non-emergency medical staff to 16-hours shifts.
• Guarantee all staff an eight-hour break between shifts.

This was later modified to allow more flexibility for non-emergency room staff but to include a limit of an average of 80 working hours per week. In addition, it was decided that nobody could reasonably be expected to work continuously for more than 24 hours.

But, at an academic level, can we assume that all doctors are seriously impaired by fatigue beyond a certain point? The evidence is very sketchy, the main problem being that the nature of the work in a hospital emergency room is often highly unpredictable. Doctors are required to assimilate the information presented by the observed symptoms and make an informed judgement on the basis of their knowledge and experience. It may well be that most of this involves straightforward deductive-type reasoning. From time to time, however, it is likely that an entirely unfamiliar and puzzling set of circumstances will arise. Simple tasks of mental arithmetic or reaction times, commonly used to assess the effects of sleep loss, can tell us little about the skills required to deal with these situations.

A small number of studies have raised specific concerns about short-term memory problems and concentration lapses. It is clear that after a night of short, frequently interrupted sleep, doctors are not able to concentrate or pay attention as well as they might normally. This is particularly the case when tasks are mundane and tedious. Junior doctors may also be impaired in their ability to learn effectively when they are extremely tired, a suggestion which clearly undermines the argument favouring the educational benefits of long hours.

At present there is no definitive study on the ability of medical professionals (or anybody else working in highly dynamic, demanding situations) to cope with day-to-day challenges following severe and acute levels of sleep loss. As is common practice with many night-shift workers, stimulants are relied on heavily, to give the impression of being wide awake. Perhaps more importantly, though, sleep loss is likely to impact on more general qualities of patient care, in which the stress of excessive sleepiness has been shown to lead to moodiness and communication difficulties: we are basically less articulate and less able to express ourselves when we are sleepy than when we are fully alert. As many studies have shown that mood effects, particularly increased irritability, are highly predictable after sleep loss, this could also have a serious impact on patient empathy. Obvious as it seems, this point tends to be under-estimated in doctor/patient relations. Doctors may simply not be as adept at sensitive consultations with patients at the end of a long shift.

Finally, there is the question of the effects of repeated sleep loss and long hours on the overall health and levels of stress for the individual doctor, a factor which is frequently given a low priority when arguments in favour of amending current practices are raised. The Libby Zion case attracted widespread publicity and has been extremely influential in shaping future policies. However, there is still considerable inertia in this area. A recent *Lancet* editorial quoted a study in which junior doctors in a major Scottish hospital regularly experienced working weeks in excess of 98 hours, with one to three hours of sleep per night being fairly routine[9]. And this despite the British government agreeing to a 72-hour maximum week for young doctors back in 1991.

Do we know when we are sleepy?

To understand how we feel at any particular point in time, especially follow-ing a disruption to our normal sleep patterns, we have to take into account the combined influence of two factors: the time of day, and how long we have been awake.

For most of us, if we get up in the morning at around 7am, by 11pm we would generally expect to be tired from the day's activities and ready for sleep. Given a sufficient incentive to stay awake, though, it would be relatively easy to carry on beyond this point, particularly with additional help – from social stimulation or caffeine, for example. By 3am we would probably be forced to rely more heavily on this additional stimulation if we were to avoid falling asleep. From this point on, the sensation of sleepiness gets progres-sively worse if sleep is delayed even further. What is perhaps surprising, however, is that by 10am the following day, after being awake for over 24 hours, the overwhelming urge to sleep would start to ease off. The reason for this is that profound sleepiness during the night results from the combined effects of an extended period without sleep and being at the circadian low point, or 'trough', in alertness. As we move into the morning phase, the effect of one of these factors (circadian-related sleepiness) is reduced, and the net effect of sleepiness becomes bearable for many people. By afternoon, how-ever, sleepiness is likely to return with a vengeance, as we move into the secondary 'dip' of the circadian cycle. We tend to find that a second night of sleep loss is beyond many people's endurance.

These two factors are very important in understanding how we feel throughout the day, and how we can predict hour-by-hour fluctuations resulting in both high and low points in alertness. It is generally assumed that an understanding of the interaction between these two influences can be used to predict the likelihood of falling to sleep at a particular point in time. This is not to say that time awake and circadian phase are the only two influences on the subjective experience of sleepiness, and considerable effort has been directed towards understanding all aspects of this state. Everyday language provides a broad range of words to describe sleepiness, but while adjectives such as 'sleepy' and 'tired' are frequently used to suggest an imme-diate desire for sleep, in certain contexts the reason for sleep is not always clear.

To convey the subtleties of how we are feeling relies on a familiarity between users based on a shared understanding of words and their meaning. Within a family, for example, word preferences, which might otherwise be misconstrued by an outside group, are used successfully to make fine distinc-tions between the various states of sleepiness. These might include the effect of a drawn-out familiar task; a long, uneventful car journey; the fatigue of personal despair and frustration; or any range of circumstances in which motivation to remain fully alert is low. Words which imply a state of sleepiness – such as lethargic, listless, drowsy, fatigued, exhausted, weary, etc – are often used to describe a specific aspect of sleepiness with may have nothing to do with the likelihood of actually falling asleep. If sleep does occur without a genuine need – for example, as a bored passenger in a car – then it is unlikely to be refreshing and will satisfy only inasmuch as it is a means of relieving boredom. On the other hand, a genuine need for sleep is understood to prompt an overwhelming desire for refreshing and revitalizing sleep.

The sensation of sleepiness plays an obvious and important role in our lives by prompting us to sleep when necessary, with the promise of restored alertness to follow. In this sense, the regularity with which we experience sleepiness serves to discipline our individual sleep habits in keeping with our bodily requirements. To confuse matters, however, it seems that we can also experience something close to sleepiness when actual sleep at that point in time is unlikely to be necessary or have any real benefit. This only becomes problematic if we need to predict the level of risk from falling asleep accidentally in a given situation.

A 'fitness to work' test

This is an ideal which, it is hoped, will help to improve the health and safety of many workers, particularly those subject to regular interruptions in sleep patterns, but not forgetting the people they are likely to come into contact with in the course of their work, whether it is other road users, patients in need of emergency care, or airline passengers. Is this a realistic goal?

There is certainly nothing new in this endeavour. In the UK, an Industrial Fatigue Research Board was set up in 1915 to counter the problems emerging from work in heavy industries and around-the-clock shift operations – problems which were to increase in subsequent years due to the demands of two prolonged periods of war. For the civilians back home, especially the women, this often involved long hours of physically demanding work. Techniques of psychological and psychometric testing were developed rapidly during this period in response to the emerging issues of work efficiency and safety, and many of the questions raised at this time are still pertinent today. For example, at what point does fatigue overwhelm? Who is most at risk? Which tasks are most likely to be affected?

From an early stage in this research, it became clear that motivation to work well would always confound the assessment of 'pure' physiological fatigue: we make similar errors through sheer boredom at the tediousness of many jobs to those we make through loss of sleep. At the other extreme, despite being extremely sleepy, there are certain tasks we are able to complete if there is sufficient incentive for us to do so. These incentives – which include fear, competition, approval-seeking and financial gain – can often, within limits, provide sufficient motivation to overcome extreme levels of tiredness.

Changes in physical measures, such as postural stability, muscle weakness, eye/hand co-ordination and manual dexterity, may not be apparent until two or three nights have passed without sleep. Clearly, these would be too insensitive in determining fitness to work. It is hoped that brain activity, particularly during the resting state, can give some indication of underlying sleepiness or, more to the point, risk of falling asleep without awareness. This has certainly been a success in diagnosing many sleep disorders, when the levels of sleepiness are extreme. But even the sleepiest person can easily be distracted for short periods, perhaps by anxiety or even heightened concern for the outcome of a test likely to have financial implications if the results point towards being unfit for work.

The current understanding of sleepiness and fatigue leaves many serious questions unanswered. As one of the most popular measures of underlying sleepiness, the speed with which a persons falls into light sleep in a quiet darkened room doesn't tell us very much about their capacity to remain awake and take part in more realistic activities. Common sense suggests that some people are simply 'good' sleepers and that the ability to fall asleep quickly at the drop of a hat is as much to do with their personal make-up as a pressing need for sleep.

So where do we draw the line? At the moment, we are not able to do this, simply because tests which pinpoint underlying levels of sleepiness (ie in the brain) are not easily reconciled with events in the real world at all levels. Unless sleepiness is extreme, it depends on exactly what it is that we are expected to do as to whether this underlying sleepiness becomes apparent as actual drowsiness or error. As already mentioned, there are many influences on the manifestation of sleepiness which need to be considered. Certain situations or repetitive tasks will almost inevitably lead to fatigue, even after a good night's sleep.

Why is sleepiness a problem?

The following is a summary of the main reasons why sleepiness may be a problem in our lives today:

• Despite limited response in light sleep, we are normally expected to remain awake during work hours. Certain occupations, particularly the military, enforce strict sanctions against falling asleep on the job.

• It is not necessary to fall asleep for an accident to happen, as more general sleepiness is also likely to reduce judgement, concentration and reaction times. But there are problems with measuring sleepiness out of context.

• A state of sleepiness or drowsiness implies that we are less than attentive – but not all jobs require 100 per cent attention. It is difficult to legislate here, although in terms of driving, most countries require a statutory obligation to at least remain attentive.

• It is possible to compensate for feeling sleepy to a limited extent, and we have no real idea how far or why some people are able to do this compared with others.

• The problem of devising shift scheduling and turnarounds is largely unresolved. Permanent nights allow some stability in sleep patterns, but the social demands are unlikely to suit many people. It is generally felt that clockwise (as opposed to anti-clockwise) shift changes are more suited to the human circadian clock, but individual differences in the ability to cope with shifts are still a puzzle, with short-sleeping 'night owls' showing the least signs of difficulty.

• Certain professions assume a unique status in the ability to compensate for the problems following sleep loss. It is interesting how we are much quicker to accept these problems in relation to commercial drivers, with obvious moves towards stricter guidelines, than we are for people in equally apparent 'life and death' situations such as the medical professions.

• A short nap (see Chapter 14) can often help, yet employers are not keen on paying people to sleep.

• The question is – are we always aware of imminent sleep and failing attentiveness? If not, then perhaps we should think more seriously about this issue before taking risks.

Chapter 14

Violence during sleep

Sleep is not always as peaceful or uneventful as we might expect. For many people, the acting out of fairly complex behaviours during sleep is a regular occurrence, with countless reports of individuals making cups of tea, preparing food or wandering round the house while sound asleep. Although most of these incidents are harmless, occasionally the consequences can be devastating. In the early hours of Sunday 24 May 1987, Kenneth Parks, a 23-year-old motor mechanic living in Toronto, Canada, drove approximately 23km (14 miles) to the home of his wife's parents, where he stabbed and killed his mother-in-law and wounded his father-in-law. There was no history of animosity between those involved and the attack was entirely unprovoked. Parks had no recollection of the entire event, which he claimed took place while he was fast asleep. When the case eventually went to trial he was acquitted of all charges for this reason[1].

Although unusual in the level of violence involved, this case was by no means the first time that the courts were asked to decide whether it is possible or even desirable to hold people legally responsible for acts of violence committed against others when they are asleep. The first detailed recording of a fatal attack dates back to the nineteenth century in Edinburgh, Scotland, when a young father, Simon Fraser, battered his infant son to death by smashing his head against a bedroom wall[2]. (There are at least two further accounts of violence during sleep in the late nineteenth century – women were involved on both these occasions, although details surrounding these cases are less well documented[3,4]). Because Fraser had a lifetime history of confused and sometimes violent behaviour during sleep, the court was sympathetic and, in the absence of legal guidelines, released him into the care of his father with an undertaking not to sleep with anybody else in the same room in the future. It is only recently, and in the advent of a number of well publicized cases, that a willingness to develop such guidelines has been shown.

The issue of responsibility during sleep is a difficult area, reflecting a complex interaction between legal, medical and popular beliefs about what we are capable of during sleep. The legal issues have tended to revolve around two factors central to the notion of guilt: a requirement for evidence of (1) an *awareness* and (2) an *intent* to carry out the criminal act in question. This poses obvious difficulties for juries, when a common experience of sleep is one in which there is little, if any, awareness of what is going on around us. On the other hand, most of us do not attack our bed partners during sleep, making it difficult for us to accept that such events are possible without some level of consciousness or prior motivation. There is also the question of whether these attacks stem from mental illness, and if so what is the likelihood of a repeat attack? Is treatment possible? Investigation of these issues has been fuelled largely by emerging medical research, which has been able to demonstrate the extent to which individuals are capable of behaving with and without awareness during sleep, highlighting genetic, physiological and environmental predisposing factors.

However, a scientific understanding of behaviours during sleep is often at odds with a more general reluctance within the population to accept the possibility of non-intentional acts of violence during sleep, and to look instead for an explanation within the context of individual incidents. These somewhat conflicting positions have made it increasingly difficult for legal systems to achieve a consistent approach.

The better known cases of violence committed against others during the course of sleep are summarized in Table 3 (opposite).

Although there is some inconsistency in rulings, on the whole it can be seen that the courts are often sympathetic to the perpetrator in these events. The victim is nearly always known to the attacker, although whether this is just because they are at hand, rather than because of some more sinister motive, is often difficult to know. More often than not, relations between attacker and victim are amicable at the time of the attack. Scientific research has been effective in contributing towards the legal debate.

Fortunately, incidences involving extreme or even fatal levels of violence during sleep are very rare. The consequences for those involved, however, can be traumatic and these seemingly senseless acts require some explanation. The most likely reaction to many of these cases is one of disbelief.

The sleeping attacker

There are a number of both general and specific questions which can help to determine whether or not an individual is genuine in claiming to have been asleep at the time of a violent attack.

What are we capable of during sleep?

Although we are often willing to accept the possibility that certain altered states of consciousness, brought about through drug use, hypnosis or even mental imbalance, can lead to behaviours which are largely beyond our control and which may not be characteristic of our normal behaviour, there is a

Table 3 **Well-known cases of violence during sleep.**

Year	Attacker	Victim	Level of violence	Outcome
1853	MINCHIN, female, England	Employee's child	Stabbed	Convicted[3]
1859	GRIGGS, female, England	Baby	Died after being thrown from window	Untried[4]
1878	FRASER, male, 33 years, Scotland	Eighteen-month-old son	Battered to death	Conditional release[2]
1949	PRICE, soldier	Male officer	Stabbed with bayonet	Acquitted[5]
1951	PALTRIDGE, male, 34 years, England	Wife	Survived axe to head	Acquitted[6]
1951	COGDEN, female, Australia	Teenage daughter	Died following blows to head with axe	Acquitted[7]
1961	BOSHEARS, male, 29 years, England	Female friend	Strangled to death	Acquitted[8]
1976	Female, 32 years, England	Husband	Stabbed but survived	Acquitted[9]
1983	Male, 14 years, Scotland	Five-year-old female cousin	Stabbed but survived	Untried[10]
1985	KEMP, England	Wife	Strangled to death	Acquitted[11]
1987	PARKS, male, 23 years, Canada	Mother-in-law, father-in-law	Mother-in-law fatally stabbed	Acquitted[1]
1991	BURGESS, male, England	Female friend	Battered but survived	Detained due to insane automatism[12]
1994	Male, 37 years, Philadelphia	Wife	Died from shotgun wound	Guilty of first-degree murder[13]

reluctance to accept that sleep is anything other than a state of relatively quiet passivity, during which we have only minimal engagement with the outside world. For many people, this is simply not the case.

Sleep-walkers have been known to drive cars to non-random destinations (as in the Parks case) and to act out familiar, routine behaviours, such as shopping and preparing food, often endangering their own safety and sometimes leading to serious or even fatal injuries through road accidents or falls. Response to pain can be also be muted during this time, meaning that sleep-walkers may not be aware of the seriousness of their own injuries, even when this involves bone fractures or life-threatening lacerations.

Sleep-walkers can also be extremely intense in pursuing their objectives, giving rise to comments about 'superhuman strength', and leading to difficulties for onlookers or potential victims who try to intervene in order to restrain them.

What are the characteristics of sleep?

As already discussed in Chapter 3, sleep is not a uniform state, but varies in a fairly predictable pattern across the night. Activity levels and responsiveness to the world about us will depend to a great extent on the state of sleep we are in at a particular time. During REM sleep, for example, although the brain would seem to be active in producing dream imagery, the body is almost completely immobilized. In contrast, NREM sleep is associated to a lesser extent with dream activity and, although we are less responsive to noise and movement in the outside world (particularly in the deeper stages of NREM sleep), the body is not immobilized to the same degree as in REM sleep. However, it is also evident that we are capable of a form of dreaming during the NREM state, without the accompanying paralysis. The distinction between REM and NREM dreams is an important one in the context of this discussion.

It is also quite normal for dreams to focus on acts of violence or aggression. A number of studies of dream content suggest that homicidal thoughts during dreaming are commonplace, although obviously these dreams are rarely acted out in real life.

Is violent behaviour during sleep part of a nightmare?

There are several different areas to consider here.

Sleep-walking, night terrors and nightmares

Sleep-walking (otherwise known as somnambulism) is the term commonly used to describe overt behaviour during sleep, in which the individual is capable of co-ordinated body movements while the brain is still firmly in a state of sleep. Most recorded cases of violence to others during sleep are considered to be examples of sleep-walking, albeit with extreme consequences.

In reality, sleep-walkers rarely imitate the rather dramatic, eyes front/arms outstretched image of the sleep-walker popularized by comedy and film. Instead, their actions can appear to be quite normal, if slightly rigid, with eyes open, but a typically blank and unresponsive facial expression. They might seem to be confused or frustrated in their actions, searching or opening doors, and if questioned will either fail to respond or give a meaningless answer. As common sense suggests, if they are in no obvious danger they should be steered gently back to bed rather than any serious attempt be made to awaken them. Most episodes of sleep-walking are not remembered on waking up in the morning.

Sleep-walking is more commonly associated with children (approximately three per cent of children are reported to experience some form of sleep-walking), and in most cases it is completely 'outgrown' by adulthood. Frequency of sleep-walking has been linked with increased levels of stress, anxiety, tiredness, etc. In children, sleep-walking can be heightened by anxiety over bed-wetting (enuresis), with confusion over finding the bathroom during this deep state of sleep. Occasionally, sleep-walking can emerge in adulthood with no prior history, and for no apparent reason.

Because of the obvious risk of self-injury, sleep-walkers have been known to devise ingenious strategies to protect themselves. These are usually geared towards keeping them within the relative safety of their bedrooms – for example, by attaching an alerting device, perhaps a bell, to the bedroom door to wake them if they try to get out.

Although the sleep-walker is not generally communicative, it is clear that they are processing incoming information to a level which allows them to perform sophisticated behaviours, such as driving a vehicle, but only with the same proficiency as during their waking life. We would not expect a novice pianist, for example, to become expert during a sleep-walking episode.

In extremely rare cases, an individual seems to be driven by malevolent impulses beyond their control, leading to physical injury or property damage. An explanation for these events in terms of acting out nightmares has some intuitive appeal. However, there are a number of facts concerning the nightmare which do not fit in with such a simple explanation.

The nightmare is a very special category of dreaming which is often thought to reflect basic personal conflicts and inner, perhaps hidden anxieties. On this level, we can identify with the terrifying and threatening nature of the nightmare and overt violent behaviours. However, we also know that the typical nightmare occurs during REM sleep, when the body is normally incapable of complex movements. There are other factors to do with the timing of most nightmares which also suggest that they are not likely to be the motivating force in violent sleep behaviours.

In the past there has been some confusion in describing the nightmare, largely because of the apparent overlap between this event and what is now described as a night terror. Although practically everybody has nightmares at some time, relatively few people experience the true night terror. While the nightmare can involve a lengthy and detailed sequence of dream events or ideas which are usually both terrifying and threatening in nature, this is generally considered to be a normal and infrequent characteristic of most people's experience of sleep. The nightmare is also generally associated with REM sleep, because of the more literal and concrete nature of the dream narrative. When we wake up from a nightmare we know almost instantly that it was just a dream. On the other hand, a night terror is often followed by a prolonged period of confusion and only semi-arousal. The night terror is also generally described in more sensational terms, such as an overwhelming feeling of being suffocated, drowned, buried or in mortal danger. Unlike the nightmare, the night terror does not involve a tangible 'storyline' to explain an overwhelming sense of dread or terror.

This type of dream is arguably more terrifying than the REM-associated nightmare, due to its being more oppressive or threatening in its nature and the delay in achieving full arousal. Night terrors are generally found to occur in NREM stages of sleep, usually during the first half of the night. This is also the period more likely to be associated with bouts of activity during sleep, and sleep-walking in particular. On waking from a night terror, individuals are frequently observed to sit bolt upright in bed with an expression of stark terror, to give out a sudden and piercing scream, and to be inconsolable in their fear. This can lead to frantic running around the room or erratic escape-type behaviours in an attempt to avoid the focus of their fear. There was some early speculation that the night terror might be some form of epileptic fit, but this was rejected when EEGs were unable to show any sign of epileptic brain activity at the time of the terror.

However, it should be noted that night terrors are by definition considered to be a separate category of sleep-related behaviour to sleep-walking, the most noticeable difference being the level of emotional arousal during a night terror, which is often accompanied by physical changes such as a rapid heartbeat and sweating. Nor is this to suggest that all violent sleep-related episodes occur outside REM sleep, as the mechanisms inhibiting movement during REM sleep can be unreliable for some individuals. There have also been reports of individuals who display complex sleep behaviours in both REM and NREM sleep. In fact, overall, the tendency for individual experiences to defy simple categorization has been one of the major obstacles to determining the source of these behaviours.

Dream enactment

In a relatively small number of instances, a bizarre and frightening dream at the time of a violent attack can be an explanatory factor. Occasionally, a history of nightmares or night terrors is also apparent in cases where individuals are involved in violent acts during sleep. However, when a nightmare is described as influencing specific acts of violence, it is nearly always in self-defence or in protection of a loved one, rather than senseless aggression.

In August 1985, a young British salesman by the name of Kemp woke up from a disturbing dream to find that his wife was dead beside him[11]. He had absolutely no recollection of causing her any harm, although there was no disputing the fact that he had strangled her. His only explanation for this act was that at the time of the attack he was in the middle of a terrifying and vivid dream in which he was being chased by Japanese soldiers armed with knives, and was forced to defend himself. There was no connection between the content of his dream and the events of his normal life, nor was there any animosity between himself and his wife to suggest a level of subconscious motivation for wanting to cause her harm. The incident was seen as an unfortunate tragedy and he was acquitted of all charges and released without condition.

In the 1950s, a middle-aged Australian woman called Mrs Cogden killed her teenage daughter as she slept in her bed, by striking her repeatedly on the head with an axe[7]. Like Kemp, she was found not guilty of murder after convincing the court that when she had delivered the fatal blows she was in fact in the middle of a dream in which she was protecting her daughter from the imminent threat of an intruder. This particular incident followed a series of related dreams, in which she imagined both herself and her daughter to be in danger. The night before the fatal attack, Mrs Cogden dreamed that the house was overrun by spiders and woke up to find herself standing over her daughter, frantically brushing imagined spiders from her face. She later recalled being visited by ghosts threatening to take her daughter away, and armed Korean soldiers besieging the house.

The influence of dreams can often provide an intuitive explanation for the level of violence in some cases, although more often than not there is no memory for either the real-life events or dream imagery. For the jury, a dream can often be the only explanation available for what might otherwise seem a senseless act.

It is interesting that the main theme in such dreams is nearly always one of self-defence following a perceived threat, and that in the mind of the attacker their actions are attempts to protect a loved one, rather than to do any harm to them.

In cases where there is a claim to have been influenced by a dream, we can never be 100 per cent certain whether the individual was asleep during the attack or, alternatively, awake but confused and disoriented by the nature of a very recent dream. The latter is believed to be the case for a number of incidents in which a person has been attacked in the process of trying to rouse somebody from sleep, when the person doing the waking is typically mistaken as a potential threat, such as an intruder. In such cases, the courts are often quite forgiving, as with the case of a young soldier by the name of Price, who stabbed and seriously wounded an officer with his bayonet[5]. The soldier described how he was in the middle of a dream when the officer tried to wake him for duty by shaking him roughly. In his half-awake state, the soldier confused this for an attack taking place in his dream, and naturally retaliated. The courts accepted his version of events and he was acquitted of malicious wounding.

Violent incidents in which there is some confusion or overlap between the dream experience and reality are in stark contrast to the Canadian case mentioned earlier, where there was no suggestion that Parks was acting under the delusion of a dream reality. Nor was Willis Boshears, when he strangled 20-year-old Jean Constable following a New Year's Eve celebration in Essex, England, in 1961[8].

At his trial, Boshears, a 29-year-old US Air Force sergeant at a local airbase, described how Ms Constable agreed to return to his flat following a New Year celebration at a local pub. A young man joined them and the three drank vodka together for the next two hours or so. At this point the young man left for home. Boshears then put a mattress in front of the fire for Ms Constable to sleep on, and fell sleep himself shortly afterwards. According to his testimony, he was next vaguely aware of being scratched around the face, only to find that when he eventually woke up Ms Constable was dead beside him. He moved her body to a bedroom and then went back to sleep in the lounge until 10am the next morning.

At the time of his subsequent arrest, he was unable to account for the scratches on his face, although it seems likely that a struggle had taken place. A neighbour remembered hearing muffled cries coming from the flat around 1am, suggesting that, if this was the time when Ms Constable was killed, Boshears had been asleep for somewhere around one to two hours.

It was to be another three days before the body was eventually found by the police, lying head first in a ditch by the side of a busy main road. It later transpired that Boshears had burned some of her clothes and removed jewellery. He was also reported to have taken a small amount of cash from her purse.

At the trial, the jury heard evidence from a pathologist expressing considerable doubts over whether it was in fact possible to strangle somebody during sleep without being wakened during the course of the attack. However, in summing up, the judge later commented on the rarity of such a defence – 'Have you ever heard of a man strangling a woman while asleep?' – and advised the jury that if they were in any doubt over whether Boshears had been completely aware of his surroundings or his capacity to take control of his actions at the time of the killing then they were obliged to acquit him. As it turned out, they had little difficulty in accepting Boshears' account, and eventually acquitted him after deliberating the evidence for less than two hours.

Timing

Most incidents of sleep-related violence occur within one to two hours of the onset of sleep. This factor can not only help to establish whether or not an individual is genuine in claiming to be asleep at the time, but is consistent with what is known about levels of arousal during sleep across the night, and particularly the distribution of REM and NREM sleep (see Chapter 3). It is not entirely clear why this should be the case, and there are notable exceptions, but there are a number of clues as to why this period of sleep is more likely to develop into a sleep-walking episode than any other.

The first one to two hours of sleep are dominated by NREM sleep, particularly the deeper Stages 3 and 4. As has previously been mentioned, the body is not immobilized in this state, and is capable of a range of fairly complex behaviours. This period is more closely associated with both sleep-walking and the occurrence of night terrors. It is also the period when it is most difficult to rouse people, when they are least likely to respond to noise or activity in the immediate environment, and when a return to full consciousness is achieved only gradually and with some confusion.

This is not to say that all sleep-related violence occurs between, for example, midnight and 2am, as shiftwork or other pressures to remain awake longer than usual often delay normal bedtimes. There is nevertheless clear evidence that the early part of sleep is a critical time in the manifestation of sleep violence.

What are the predisposing factors to identify individuals at risk?

There have been a number of attempts to identify factors which are likely to predispose an individual to activity during sleep which may endanger themselves or others. As these typically involve the retrospective study of individuals who have presented themselves at a medical centre, either under their own volition or through spousal or family pressure, it is often very difficult to get some measure of the prevalence of these types of behaviours in the more general population. For example, in many of the cases cited, the individuals would typically have dealt with problems related to this behaviour for many years without expert help, only turning to medical advice as a last resort or following personal injury. Some interesting factors have come to light as a result of these investigations:

• There is a strong tendency for sleep-walking and night terrors to run in families.
• A combination of sleep-walking and night terrors is far more likely to occur in men than in women.
• The first experience of this can emerge in adulthood and is not necessarily a development from childhood sleep-walking.
• The vast majority of sleep-walkers show no signs of abnormal behaviour during their waking life. This point is particularly interesting, because until recently it was assumed that sleep-walking was symptomatic of underlying emotional difficulties.
• The onset of these behaviours can be linked to life events, especially those associated with post-traumatic stress disorder.
• Only very occasionally is sleep-walking related to damage to the brain (through accident or disease).

In nearly all cases, it is reported that people at risk from injury to themselves or others during sleep have some combination of the above factors as part of their individual make-up.

What are the circumstances leading up to an incident?

There has been considerable emphasis on the circumstances leading up to a violent incident during sleep. For individuals who are predisposed, these factors may acts as triggers to acts of violent. Stress and anxiety are frequently cited as important factors in this respect. This link was first described around the time of World War II, when returning soldiers, haunted by the images of the war, would wake up suddenly and 'fight' off attacks from imaginary enemy soldiers. Nowadays, these soldiers would probably be described as suffering from post-traumatic stress disorder, and would be offered psychological or pharmacological help in dealing with their anxieties.

In the search for an explanation for otherwise meaningless and senseless acts of violence, investigators have looked for evidence of stressful experiences, such as recent disagreements or ongoing relationship difficulties, which could account, even at a subconscious level, for the violent behaviour. A particularly perplexing example of this was the case of a 14-year-old boy who stabbed and seriously wounded his five-year-old cousin as she slept[10]. There was no obvious explanation for this behaviour: the boy had never displayed an aggressive or violent tendency, he got on well with his cousin, and was generally considered to be well balanced in his emotional outlook. He had no recollection of the attack, and only became aware of it after the alarm was raised, at which point he woke up in one of the downstairs rooms of the house.

During the course of the investigation, it became clear that the boy had some emotional difficulties, although these might be considered relatively minor and fairly normal for his age. He did not get on with his father, and, throughout the evening of the attack, he was described by his aunt as being in a fairly unhappy mood following an argument with friends. A psychiatric report, instrumental in securing his release without charge, described him as being angry on going to sleep. The importance of his mood at this point is unclear, however, although in combination with a previous history of fairly animated sleep talking and gesturing, it may have been the key to the subsequent attack.

Disruption to normal sleep patterns, leading to acute sleep deprivation or interrupted sleep, has also been identified as an important issue, and is thought to be related directly to the frequency of sleep-walking events. The reasons for this are not clear, but reduction in sleep quality and quantity immediately prior to a sleep-walking incident is likely to result in deeper sleep during the early stages of the night, reduced response to environmental events, resistance to attempts at being woken, and increased confusion on waking. This is likely to be exacerbated further by long-term alcohol use and unfamiliar sleeping arrangements, factors which have also been found to be important in some cases. In the Boshears case, for example, the attack occurred following an evening of drinking (it was New Year's Eve) and after both Boshears and his victim had fallen asleep in a makeshift bed on the living-room floor of his flat.

But this does not explain why most people are able to tolerate normal everyday stresses such as these without their unwelcome intrusion into sleep.

Is there always a full memory of an event?

The importance of whether or not there is a memory of an event is a point on which researchers have disagreed. During sleep, we do not normally expect to register what is happening in the real world to any great extent, and a literal memory for the factual details is unlikely to convince a jury that the attacker was actually asleep at the time. It is far more likely that certain aspects of the attack (positioning of the hands, etc) infiltrate a powerful dream. On the other hand, most attackers have absolutely no recollection of the event, and are deeply traumatized to discover the consequences of their actions on waking.

What is the normal 'waking' relationship with the injured party?

Not all juries are willing to accept that violence during sleep is completely unmotivated and beyond the control of an attacker, particularly when the relationship between attacker and victim comes under suspicion. There are no recorded cases of sleep-related violence towards complete strangers, although this may be because most attacks occur in the bedroom where strangers are simply less available.

The relationship between attacker and victim had a significant bearing on the outcome of a recent case in Philadelphia, in which a 37-year-old man was charged with the fatal shooting of his wife[13]. He described having no memory for the event and claimed that he must have been asleep as he reached under the bed for the gun and then shot his wife at point-blank range. The man had a diagnosed sleep condition which, although not usually associated with sleep violence, meant that his sleep was severely disrupted throughout the whole of the night. His defence team argued that as the cumulative effects of this condition on long-term sleep disruption leads to overwhelming and pro-found sleepiness throughout the day, this would make him a likely candidate for sleep-walking and night terrors (particularly as he had been known to sleep-walk as a child). However, there was no medical evidence to establish a link between his specific condition and violence during sleep.

In this particular case, there were also a number of other factors to under-mine the credibility of the defendant's account. The shooting took place approximately one hour after he claimed to have fallen asleep, which is consistent with the placement of many night terrors related to NREM sleep. However, the recording of his emergency call showed him to be lucid and calm, even though the call was allegedly made within minutes of him waking and discovering his wife's body. There was little sign of confusion or emotional distress, as might normally be expected. Although he was to eventually describe a hunting dream coinciding with the shooting, in his earlier statements he claimed to have no recollection of a dream that night.

On the other hand, it is likely that the jury were more interested in the accounts of friends and family members, who described his long history of waking hostility and violence towards his wife and told how she had plans to leave her husband in the near future. He was eventually convicted of first-degree murder and sentenced to life imprisonment.

Often, the more unlikely the target for violence, the greater the possibility of having a sympathetic response to a claim to have been asleep at the time of the attack. In the case of Paltridge, for example, which took place in England in 1951, a wife actually testified in court in support of her husband after surviving a sleep-walking attack in which he struck her with an axe[7]. In another extraordinary case in the 1970s, a 32-year-old housewife and mother from Preston, England, was found not to be legally responsible for stabbing her husband as he slept. The court heard how she had woken up during the night and, finding it difficult to return to sleep, had gone down to the kitchen to peel potatoes for the following day. She later returned to her bed, which she shared with her husband, and went back to sleep. Between this point and eventually being woken at around 8am by her distressed husband, she had managed to stab him over 15 times in the chest and back with the potato peeler. When the case eventually came to court, the jury heard that despite extensive medical and psychological enquiries, no explanation for this attack had been possible. The accused woman, who was supported by her husband throughout the trial, described her ten-year marriage as happy and stable, and could offer no explanation for what had happened that night. Given the nature of their relationship, the judge considered the attack to be an involuntary action, entirely out of character with the woman's normal waking behaviour.

Eight years later, the consultant psychiatrist at the time of the trial wrote to the *British Journal of Psychiatry* by way of an update[9]. He reported that there had been no recurrence of sleep-related violence towards the husband and that the couple remained happily married.

What is the behaviour on waking from a violent event?

Most people have described their absolute horror on waking to find that they have seriously or perhaps even fatally injured a loved one during their sleep. With a few notable exceptions, this seems to be the more normal reaction for the cases that have been investigated, and the one expected by jurors. Following the guilty verdict in the Philadelphia shotgun murder in 1994, there was some speculation in the American press concerning the jury's disapproval of the husband's behaviour on discovering his wife's body. It may be that he came across as 'too unmoved' by the events, as evidenced by the clarity of his call to the emergency services, and his lack of inclination to stem the flow of blood or provide first aid assistance for his injured wife.

Not all juries have been this critical, however. The Boshears jury, for example, was surprisingly forgiving of his behaviour after the discovery of Jean Constable's body, finding nothing unusual about the idea of him going back to sleep for a further six hours despite the realization that he had probably killed her, or the great lengths that he went to in order to dispose of the body and other incriminating evidence.

A legal responsibility

As can be seen from Table 3 on page 185, the courts are often reluctant to punish individuals who have committed serious, even fatal, acts of aggression against others, if it can be shown that they were asleep at the time of the act. In order for them to be held legally responsible for such crimes, it has been necessary to show that the individual was both aware and in control of their actions throughout. We have only recently seen the development of guidelines more specific to the question of sleep-walking as, historically, the case law in this area is disjointed and somewhat inconsistent. This may have led to the more general perception that sleep-walking incidents are too rare to warrant any special legal provision. For example, in the Boshears case the judge asked the jury: 'Have you ever heard of a man strangling a woman while asleep? Does there exist any record that such things happen?' Press reporting of this case, and perhaps some surprise over the outcome, prompted a discussion in the House of Lords over the need for a change in the law. However, it was again decided that the circumstances of the case were so unusual as to be unlikely to occur again, and the suggestion was rejected.

In many of the cases brought to trial, the decision has been that the behaviour during sleep constitutes a form of 'automatism', a state which precludes intentional or willed action. However, 'automatism' is a legal rather than a medical concept. It is not limited to acts of sleep-walking, and can also cover reduced awareness due to epileptic fits, insulin imbalance, drug intake and carbon monoxide poisoning.

This position was made clear in 1961, in the case of Bratty, a young Irishman charged with the murder of a young girl after offering her a lift home in his car one night[14]. At his trial, Bratty gave a vivid and detailed account of strangling the young girl to death with her own stocking, before driving to a secluded spot in the road and pushing her body out of the car. Throughout the entire episode he described being overcome with a 'terrible feeling and then a sort of blackness'. His defence argued (unsuccessfully) that he had suffered an epileptic seizure at the time of the attack and that, as he was unable to control his actions, he could not be held accountable. The case went to appeal at the House of Lords, where Lord Denning made what was to be an extremely influential statement concerning the legal status of acts committed during a state of automatism (note the reference to sleep-walking):

> No act is punishable if it is done involuntarily: and an involuntary act in this context – some people nowadays refer to it as 'automatism' – means an act which is done by the muscles without any control by the mind, such as a spasm, a reflex action or a convulsion; or an act done whilst suffering from concussion or whilst sleep-walking.

Note that until the 1980s, however, the courts showed little concern for the medical explanation of sleep-walking, relying instead on a more common-sense understanding of this behaviour. It is only recently, with the introduction of testimony from 'expert' witnesses (usually specialists from the sleep disorders field) to provide credence to both prosecution and defence arguments, that these issues have been considered. The medical position is now considered to be central to most cases.

Is the violent sleep-walker mentally ill?

The notion of automatism can be further sub-divided into (1) non-insane and (2) insane automatism. Until recently, cases where sleep-walking is accepted and defined as an act of automatism were invariably assigned to the non-insane category. The main difference for the accused is that while a finding of 'not guilty' due to non-insane automatism automatically secures their release, 'not guilty' through insane automatism requires that they be detained indefinitely for psychiatric assessment and possible treatment. In the state of insane automatism, the individual is presumed to be influenced by a 'disease of the mind' and in need of medical help, even though this may refer to a momentary state which is unlikely to recur. Both positions accept the involuntary nature of the act; however, they also say something about the normality of such an occurrence, which, particularly in the case of sleep-walking, has only recently been addressed through a number of difficult cases.

The question of the mental status of an individual at the time of a sleep-walking attack was first explored in any depth in the case of Parks, in which he was acquitted of the murder and serious wounding of his in-laws. In this case, expert witnesses were called upon to offer an opinion as to Parks' mental status at the time of the attack. In particular, a number of specialist sleep-disorder clinicians testified against the likelihood of him suffering from a mental disorder and Parks was subsequently released without condition.

A similar discussion was to take place shortly afterwards in the British courts. In this case the accused, a young man by the name of Burgess, was charged with wounding with intent to do grievous bodily harm[12]. The court was told how Burgess attacked a young female friend with a glass bottle and a video cassette recorder, before attempting to throttle her. There had been no previous animosity between the pair. Burgess had invited the young woman to spend the evening at his flat, during the course of which they each drank a single glass of martini and watched the television together, before falling asleep on the settee. The woman then remembered waking up around an hour and a half later to find Burgess's hands around her throat. He appeared to her to be asleep or in a trance-like state, although she was eventually able to wake him with her struggles and he released his grip immediately. The young woman had a head wound (apparently from being hit by a bottle and the video recorder), but did not remember being hit.

Although Burgess had no memory of the attack, he showed considerable remorse and wrote an apologetic letter to his victim in which he explained: 'I must have had some kind of blackout or fit'. But he also hinted that it was not entirely unexpected and that he was concerned with the state of his own mind: 'I have known for some time that I was heading for some sort of breakdown'.

The decision of the court was that Burgess was not guilty of the offence by reason of insane automatism. This case was unusual, in that for the first time sleep-walking was designated to be a pathological condition – 'a disease of the mind' which required indefinite detention for medical treatment. An appeal was lodged, but in maintaining the original ruling, Lord Lane pointed out that, with the exception of the Parks case, this was perhaps the first occasion on which the courts had had the 'advantage' of expert knowledge in the area of sleep behaviours.

These cases have prompted considerable legal discussion, not least because of the important differences in thinking between expert witnesses. At the Parks trial, sleep-walking was described by invited specialists as normal, if unusual, behaviour and not to be considered in any way pathological, whereas experts in the Burgess trial testified that sleep-walking was in fact an abnormal mental condition for which treatment was necessary.

What is the level of awareness during sleep?

Awareness is rarely clear cut in relation to sleep and wakefulness – we can drift into an objectively defined brain state of sleep, and yet still retain the ability to respond to aspects of our environment. Even in the deepest stages of sleep (Stages 3 and 4), we are responsive to highly personal information (we can show this by whispering the sleeper's name into their ear), suggesting that we still 'hear' during sleep, albeit at a very selective level. We also find that the transition between wake and sleep (in both directions) is rarely abrupt, and that we are more likely to show a waxing and waning between states as we go to sleep and wake up. This can be more intense when there is some conflict between the two states – for example, if we are not really ready to wake up (particularly in the middle of the night) or if we try to sleep when there is no urgent need. Awareness can also be distorted by drugs, alcohol and anaesthesia. When we describe somebody as being asleep, it is tempting to assume that this is synonymous with a total lack of awareness, whereas this is not always the case and can be very misleading (particularly if being asleep is central to a defence argument).

What is the potential for willed or controlled action during sleep?

With this in mind, not everybody is convinced that we are totally oblivious to our surroundings when we are asleep, or that we are incapable of responding to them. In a recent report, a Canadian psychiatrist, Dr Peter Roper, gave the example of a case in which he had treated a young, female habitual sleep-walker prone to excessive binge eating during her nocturnal wanderings[15]. Having discovered that the young woman had a phobia about snakes, Dr Roper was able to turn this to his advantage by each night using a toy snake to block the path to the refrigerator door. Whenever the snake was in place, no attempt was made to get to the food inside the fridge, despite the fact that the woman was sleep-walking at the time. Her husband added that she only ever returned to her old habits on the few occasions when he had forgotten to put the snake in place before going to bed.

Dr Roper argued that the success of this rather novel treatment was because the woman was still able to register the significance of the snake barring her way even though she was probably in a deep state of sleep. The fact that she was reluctant to walk past the snake suggests she was acting on information processed during sleep, and, in effect, making a considered decision on the basis on that information.

This case suggests that, despite conventional wisdom, the sleep-walker is capable of taking things in, and that their actions are not entirely without reason or control. Of course, it is practically impossible to say, from one person to another, and from one sleep-walking episode to another, just how much awareness and control a person may have. It does seem likely, though, that it is not quite such an 'all or nothing' situation as the courts have implied in the past.

Is premeditation during dreaming proof of intent?

In the recent and very well-publicized O.J. Simpson trial, in which the celebrity was accused of the murder of his wife, Nicole Brown, and her friend, Ronald Goldman, the presiding judge, Judge Lance Ito, made what was for some the astonishing move of allowing testimony to be presented before the court which related to the contents of O.J. Simpson's dreams. Having successfully argued the point that dreams have elements of 'wish-fulfilment', the prosecution were allowed to submit evidence from a Mr Ronald Shipp, who described a conversation in which, a short time after the murders, O.J. Simpson told him: 'To be truthful Ron, I have had a lot of dreams about killing her'.

The prosecution was no doubt relying on the popular belief that at the centre of all dreams is an element of truth. This was an idea introduced by Freud (see Chapter 2) and is readily accepted at a popular level. Yet, as Freud himself recognized, the adult dream is a complex construction, involving much symbolism and hidden meaning. It is unusual to expect the dream to provide a simple statement of intent, as is suggested here. Many dreams are very odd indeed, and it is an alarming suggestion that we might be expected to defend them in a court of law. The level of brutality in dreams as a whole has been found to be extremely high but, as previously noted, there is little to suggest any genuine motivation or desire to act out this violence. On this basis, the dream is hardly a safe and reliable construct for inclusion in a legal context, as its relation with reality is still so poorly understood.

A continuing danger

Finally, there is the question of how to deal with these violent events in the longer term.

What is the likelihood of recurrence?

The question of continuing danger (either to himself or others) was a fundamental consideration in the case of Parks. The court heard from experts that it was highly unlikely that he would attack anybody in the future in similar circumstances, and that consequently there was only minimal risk in releasing Parks without medical or psychiatric treatment. When the case came to the Canadian Supreme Court, however, there was some disagreement between judges on this issue. It was suggested that the likelihood of recurrence could be even further reduced through improved sleep 'hygiene' techniques (ie to maintain a more regular sleep pattern and avoid periods of acute sleep loss), although the courts were not able to impose this restriction with the legal procedures at their disposal.

Since this trial, the Canadian government has proposed statutory amendments to the effect that in future cases of this kind it would be possible to impose such restrictions following a similar verdict. Within the same white paper, it has also been proposed that the distinction in automatism along the lines of mental illness is no longer necessary or appropriate in respect of sleep-walking. Instead, cases of automatism would be considered for post-trial treatment (custodial if necessary) where appropriate. This has the advantage of providing the option of a discretionary treatment order without the need to categorize a sleep-walker as being mentally ill.

Although many people experience sleep-walking and night terrors throughout their lives, there is no reason to expect escalation in the intensity of such behaviour. Reassuringly, there have been no reported cases involving a recurrence of extreme violence.

Is medical treatment necessary or available?

When an individual has been considered to be at serious risk, perhaps through repeated self-injuries, a number of pharmacological treatments have been found to be effective in preventing sleep-walking. For the chronic sleep-walker, the situation is likely to be improved by avoiding stress where possible, as well as acute disruption to normal sleeping patterns. It is not known whether this approach would have been effective or even appropriate for many of the cases discussed. While there is evidence in some instances of a prior history, this was not the case for the Boshears or Burgess cases, where the violent sleep behaviours came totally out of the blue.

The questions remain

It is clear that in both medical and legal contexts there are still many issues to be resolved concerning sleep-related behaviours. There are also a number of puzzling factors. For example, why it is that most of these cases involve men? Why is the mode of violence nearly always described as protective (either of themselves or loved ones), when 'everyday' violence is just as likely to be motivated by territoriality, sexuality and greed? There is no clear picture as to how important experiences of this kind are in motivating the individual to engage in a physical attack.

There is some anecdotal evidence to suggest that for some people the act of violence is the physical realization of a threat manifested within a nightmare (they are literally acting out their dream), but this is not always the case. For a substantial proportion of extremely brutal, often fatal attacks, the attacker has absolutely no recollection of the event and displays none or very few of the factors predisposing an individual towards these behaviours.

Chapter 15

Too busy to sleep?

T here have been many experimental attempts to explore the boundaries of human sleep need by exposing willing volunteers to quite extreme deviations from a normal sleep pattern. Much of this work was designed to show how little sleep an individual could endure without serious risk, whether over the long or short term. The findings from such 'marathon' periods without sleep appear to be at odds with the contemporary understanding of sleep need as somewhere in the region of eight hours per night for the average individual. However, the main thrust of these early studies was to explore the risk of serious or permanent injury following total sleep loss or dramatically reduced sleep. Over the last ten years or so there has been a growing awareness of what some have called an 'epidemic' of sleeplessness across the western world, the effects of which are often underestimated or played down as a result of a more general preoccupation with industrious activity at all costs.

Various recent estimates in the popular press in the USA report that over a half of all Americans are not getting enough sleep, for one reason or another. With similar claims in many other areas of the world, such concerns are currently high on the scientific agenda. As few people complain of sleeping too much, a widespread sense of insufficient sleep has been linked with the problems of living in a more complex society and is often compared, rather nostalgically, with a period not so long ago when demands on time were presumed to be fewer. However, records are scarce, and we know little with any certainty about 'pre-industrialization' sleep habits.

Living round the clock

Research emphasis has nevertheless undergone a distinct shift towards a more pragmatic approach to studying the effects of sleep loss. It is relatively unlikely that many of us will ever have to deal with the effects of 11 consecutive nights without sleep. On the other hand, there are occupations for which a single night without sleep is common. What is it about living in a modern age that acts as an imperative to avoid sleep? Three areas take special blame: work, leisure and sleep disorders.

We have seen in recent years a massive increase in the number of reported diagnosis of disorders of night-time sleep which impact on daytime alertness; this is especially the case for sleep apnoea and insomnia, for example. We also rely more than ever before on artificial aids, such as caffeine and prescribed sleeping pills, to 'manage' sleep and wake at our convenience. Shiftwork and trans-global travel make additional demands on the body's natural sleep rhythm.

Many of these trends are intimately linked with changes in the way we work: more people work from home, or work flexible hours, rotating shifts or throughout the night than ever before. In the USA, it has been estimated that over half the adult population work outside the traditional nine to five business hours at some point during their working lives. As the distinction between day and night is obscured for an increasing range of activities, we may wonder whether we are moving towards a society which is simply too busy to sleep?

For many areas of the service and retail industries, traditional business hours have been replaced by an 'open all hours' approach, with retailers and financiers recognizing the advantages of being able to offer total flexibility, including the convenience of relatively 'hassle-free' transactions during off-peak hours. By providing the ultimate in round-the-clock availability, 24-hour services are definitely here to stay. It is now possible to do the weekly shopping, pay bills, check bank balances, book holidays, arrange insurance and mortgages, and visit the cinema, museum or restaurant at practically any hour of the day or night. In the home, a steady flow of television and radio programmes, instant global communications, caffeine and electric lighting all conspire to keep us awake.

The physical boundaries between work and leisure are also blurring, with a move away from office-based work. E-mail, Internet communications, lap-top computers and so on have all helped in transforming the office to a 'virtual' concept for many people, where the boss, thanks to networking facilities, can literally be looking over your shoulder wherever you may be working. Rather than liberating, this can have the paradoxical effect of increasing availability for work, on a 24-hours, seven-days-a-week basis if and when the job demands.

Night working has always been an essential, if unpopular, obligation for occupations which need to provide 24-hour cover for emergency or security, or to keep expensive industrial plants in continuous operation. The difficulties with working at a time when the body normally expects to be asleep are well recognized: low productivity, high accident rate, absenteeism, and even long-term health problems. Shiftworkers also experience major social problems, as they sleep and wake out of synchrony with the rest of the family, and will often find themselves trying to sleep during the day, when the world outside their bedroom window is bustling with activity. Over the years many different patterns of shift 'rotation' have been advocated in an attempt to master such problems, and legislative bodies have always been active in this area to provide protection for those involved.

The effects of social pressures to postpone sleep in favour of more active nocturnal pursuits have been linked with an increase in traffic accidents (see Chapter 13), more fatigue during the day, work and educational problems, irritability and lack of drive. A number of major accidents and 'near misses' have been associated with poor sleep habits, with many people calling for radical changes to the way sleep is prioritized in a modern world.

As the demand for maximum availability is met, shiftwork is now a reality for a vast number of occupations, with enthusiasm for all-night electronic call centres accounting for a drastic change in work practices over recent years, particularly for women. In the UK, it is currently estimated that more than a million people work between the hours of 9pm and 6am on a regular basis. In the near future, it will no longer be appropriate to speak in terms of 'unsociable hours' for the shiftworker, as the nocturnal lifestyle is becoming more of a reality for large sections of our society.

However, shiftwork can lead to long-term problems, and is linked with higher rates of gastrointestinal and cardiovascular disease, stress and mood-related disorders. Many of the subjective problems stem from difficulty in sleeping between shifts, especially during daytime hours, when there are numerous distractions and the body is least likely to demand sleep. The social significance of long-term shiftwork tends to be downplayed in relation to physiological concerns, yet lack of contact with family members, the effects of irritability on social relations, and erratic leisure hours compound further the physiological difficulties of shiftwork. The immediate family also suffers (albeit indirectly) from the bad moods, lethargy and excessive fatigue experienced by the shiftworker out of work hours.

Night workers also tend to revert to a night-time sleeping pattern on their days off, mainly to accommodate their domestic and social interests, but perhaps also because of the ongoing difficulties with sleeping during the day. For those working on rotating shifts, the problem is compounded by regular changes in sleep arrangements so that the body never completely adapts to the imposition of an artificial routine. Experimentation with rescheduling light treatment to 'fool' the brain into an inverted day/night has shown some success in this area. When to eat is an additional problem for the shiftworker, with daytime fasting and night-time eating often mismatched with the physiological needs of the body.

Do things get better over time? The problems experienced by shiftworkers are a combination of long-term sleep restriction, inappropriate sleep times in relation to circadian factors, and social and psychological stress. Unfortunately, normal age-related changes in sleep patterns may add to these difficulties.

To sum up, there are currently genuine concerns that we are moving too far away from our natural pattern of activity, and that this may have detrimental effects in the long run. So is society really anti-sleep?

Alarm clocks

In an ideal world, sleep should be allowed to come to its natural conclusion, or so the argument goes. The fact that the vast majority of people use alarm clocks to wake up in the morning, rather than leaving it to chance, is often considered to be a significant indication of insufficient sleep. On weekends and holidays, when alarm clocks are more likely to be abandoned, we sleep an extra hour or so each morning. Using an alarm clock during the week suggests that perhaps we are (1) sleeping heavily due to acute sleep loss and (2) forcing ourselves to wake up before we are ready. On the other hand, is there any reason to assume that waking up naturally will always coincide with the satiation of a biological need for sleep? The most obvious reason for relying so extensively on alarm clocks to wake us in the morning is that we simply cannot rely on our own internal 'clock' if it is important for us to be up by a certain time. But some people claim to know the time during sleep and will automatically wake up a few minutes before the alarm goes off.

This possibility was put to the test in the early 1980s at the San Jose State University in the USA[1]. The aim of this study was to ask whether volunteers who considered themselves good at waking unaided could do this at any point in the night (ie as if they really did keep track of time), and not just close to their normal wake times (which suggests more of a habit). One hundred and fifty undergraduate students took up this challenge and chose for themselves eight convenient nights on which to try out their skill at 'self-awakening' on cue. On half the nights, a target time was agreed which was roughly one hour after lights out. On the other four nights, the target time was set at one hour before normal wake times. Volunteers were instructed to turn off the lights as usual and attempt to sleep until waking spontaneously, the idea being that they should 'will' themselves to wake up at the pre-agreed time. If they did wake up during the night, then they were only to look at a clock and record the time if they were convinced that it was reasonably close to the time of their intended waking. Not surprisingly, volunteers had more success (about a 60 per cent hit rate) with the second condition – waking up an hour before their normal morning wake-up time. Even so, they still managed to wake up close to the early waking times (an hour after going to bed) on about half the attempts.

This difference between early and later awakenings was anticipated by the experimenters for a number of reasons. Not only is an hour after falling asleep the least familiar time for waking up, but normal sleep continuity suggests a more profound state of sleep during the early part of the night.

This would almost definitely have made the volunteers less responsive to the environment during this half of the night, and more sleepy on waking.

What was perhaps even more interesting, though, was that the most successful volunteers overall, who showed a clear talent for waking up at a pre-determined time, described themselves as generally poor sleepers. Although poor sleepers were not exceptionally good at the earlier awakenings, there was a clear difference between them and sounder sleepers for the late awakenings. This suggests that being able to wake up before the alarm in the morning, as many people claim, is more to do with an increase in spontaneous awakenings as the night draws to a close. The fact that eventually one of these awakenings also happens to occur at a time when we have 'chosen' to wake up may be largely due to coincidence, rather than an internal 'timekeeping' mechanism.

Towards the end of sleep, we tend to keep a close check on what is happening around us and use these clues to monitor time on an almost subconscious level. In a normal environment, we soon become familiar with changes that coincide with the start of the day – traffic noise, light, heating and more general activity levels. We are so good at this that we often remember waking up slightly before the alarm, in anticipation of it going off.

So why do we need an alarm clock? Is it because we are not getting enough sleep (and insist on waking up before we are truly refreshed), or is it simply because we are not very good at waking up when we want to? In this study, the experimenters considered a self-awakening to be a 'success' if volunteers were within 30 minutes of the target time. This would hardly be considered a practical success in real terms, where arriving at work on time every day is important, and half an hour can make all the difference.

Can we reasonably expect to manage without an alarm clock? Some people can do it some of the time – but they will occasionally, and for no obvious reason, be let down. Will sleeping longer improve on this level of accuracy and reliability? This has never been shown experimentally, although more sleep at night does lead to more brief awakenings during the second half of the night. It may be that sleep gets more difficult as we sleep longer nights, in that sleep is lighter and more prone to disturbance towards the morning, but there is no good reason to expect time-keeping, as in the ability to wake up at a pre-set time, to improve as a result.

Caffeine

Caffeine is probably the most popular legal, non-prescribed stimulant in the world. The daily consumption of caffeinated food products and beverages, such as tea, coffee, soft drinks and chocolate, has increased enormously over the last 100 years or so. So do we rely on caffeine all too often as a poor substitute for sleep?

Addiction and long-term health problems are the two main worries for caffeine consumers, with many now preferring non-caffeinated or de-caffeinated alternatives. It is not always easy to gauge just how much caffeine is being consumed; a single cup of coffee contains widely varying amounts of caffeine, and strength of flavour may not be a reliable indication of this. Laboratory studies looking into the effects of caffeine have produced many inconsistencies, although the short-term behavioural effects of moderate doses appear to be harmless for most people. On the other hand, the addictive properties of caffeine are poorly understood and rely to a great extent on individual tolerance. Caffeine is excellent at reducing fatigue, whether it is due to genuine sleepiness or just boredom or monotony.

Beneficial effects on cognitive performance are doubtful, although an improvement in feeling alert is likely to lead to increased motivation to apply more effort or pay more attention to a task. Most of the laboratory tests on the effects of caffeine have used volunteers who are already presumed to have had enough sleep. Despite feeling more awake from taking caffeine, there are no benefits to short-term memory, for example. The effects of caffeine on what might be called 'high-level' decision-making are also unclear, although insofar as caffeine increases motivation and reduces fatigue there may be some indirect benefit. But too much caffeine can lead to over-arousal and distraction, an effect which may depend on personality type. This has been demonstrated for introverts and extroverts, the former becoming 'over-aroused' and showing a decline in performance with smaller amounts of caffeine than the latter. The suggestion is that extroverts have lower 'background' levels of arousal than introverts, and are therefore able to tolerate more stimulation from artificial sources, such as caffeine. Although the idea that extroverts are under-aroused may seem a contradiction in terms, it has been argued that a constant zest for activity and social stimulation signifies a compensatory mechanism for this presumed under-stimulation. But this effect also depends on the time of day – extroverts benefit most from caffeine in the morning, and introverts in the evening.

Certainly, caffeine consumption is habit-forming. It is an easy 'fix' and the subjective effects are quite strong, and probably more noticeable the more fatigued we are at the time of consumption. This is especially the case first thing in the morning or last thing at night, when we insist in staying up to finish something off before going to bed.

Can we do without caffeine? It seems so. When volunteers are denied access to caffeinated coffee and offered 'de-caff' substitutes, their consumption (in cups per day) falls over the first few days. After this initial period, however, they gradually develop a taste for de-caff to the same level as their previous caffeinated coffee habit. This suggests that there is a strong force of habit with coffee drinking, perhaps reinforced by social conditions, that is not entirely dependent on its stimulating properties. Yet withdrawal from early-morning caffeine can be a problem in the early stages, with headaches, listlessness and difficulty in getting started all blamed on an abrupt denial of this post-sleep 'fix'.

But are we so dosed up with caffeine that we forget what it feels like to be wide awake through natural processes? There are some contradictions here. Many people claim to get most benefit from caffeine first thing in the morning and perhaps this does suggest that we could really do with more sleep. But why do we expect to wake up feeling refreshed and alert? It takes quite some time to shift from wake to sleep when we go to bed at night: about 20 minutes normally, and five to ten if we are very sleepy. Is there, then, any reason to expect an abrupt shift between waking and sleep at the other end of the night? A certain amount of difficulty in getting moving is probably quite normal. This may be even more drawn out the longer we have spent asleep: a 'lie in' of an extra one to two hours at the weekend can take some shaking off. On the other hand, when it is important for us to get moving – and many people like to cut things fine – a strong cup of coffee is a convenient way of 'kick-starting' the day if you haven't the time to come round more naturally.

Perhaps the biggest concern is really with late-night caffeine consumption. It is at this time that the effects of caffeine are often under-estimated, and even early-evening coffee-drinking can interfere with a good night's sleep. For those people who are already experiencing problems with sleep, caffeinated beverages should definitely be avoided. There is also considerable parental concern over the high levels of caffeine in popular soft drinks and chocolate products. One of the problems with this is that caffeine has such as strong association with coffee, and little else, that we may not realize just how much is being consumed by children on a regular daily basis.

Of course, for adults there may be circumstances when it is simply not convenient or even safe to sleep. Under these conditions, caffeine or other artificial stimulants have their uses. But these situations should be avoided as far as possible. Caffeine can give the impression that fatigue is under control, when it fact this may not be the case. It is likely to alter judgement over whether you are in a suitable condition to drive a car, for example. Finally, caffeine can never be an adequate substitute for sleep: the alerting effects are superficial and an urge for sleep will undoubtedly return with a vengeance. If coffee is needed in large doses to keep going at the end of the day, this is a strong hint from the body that it is time to sleep.

Sleeping pills

What about the other extreme – needing to sleep when the body is either not willing or able to co-operate? It has been estimated that as much as 25 per cent of the population suffer some form of insomnia, ie difficulty in getting to sleep or sleeping throughout the night. These problems increase with age, with older women in particular being more likely to admit to have difficulties in sleeping than men. Sleep problems often emerge at a time of particular life stress, including marital breakdown, bereavement, job loss, ill health, etc, although occasionally the ability to sleep soundly breaks down for no obvious reason.

For many, the problems can be short term and a number of remedies are on hand to deal with these difficulties. Alcohol has always been a popular choice. However, although moderate amounts can help with falling to sleep, alcohol has quite a strong disruptive effect on the rest of the night, thereby interfering with the overall restorative properties of sleep (see Chapter 5). There are also many over-the-counter 'soporifics' which some find useful, although anything stronger is usually only available on medical prescription.

The consumption of sleeping pills is currently at an all-time high, with an ongoing commitment from pharmaceutical companies to develop newer and more effective drugs, with fewer side effects. Repeat prescribing without review by medical examination is also a common practice in distributing sleeping pills. Modern sleeping pills can be very effective in helping people to fall asleep faster and/or improving the continuity of sleep throughout the night, leading to an increased perception of good quality sleep. However, they have also been associated with undesirable side effects, the most difficult of which usually centre on feelings of fatigue and lethargy throughout the following day. This can only add to the difficulties experienced by shiftworkers, who rely more heavily on sleeping pills than fixed-shift day workers.

Common sense suggests that sleeping pills are most useful for the more transient sleep difficulty, often in relation to a major life event or disruption. But it is also common for them to be prescribed when sleep problems are secondary or symptomatic of an underlying psychological difficulty, such as a depressive illness. This is particularly true for the elderly, who have the additional problem of coming to terms with age-related changes in sleep patterns. Alternatives to treating insomnia with sleeping pills are available, including behaviour or cognitive modifications, an example of which was described in Chapter 4. In this case, weekly television broadcasts covering advice and education about the importance of maintaining regular daily habits and realistic expectations about how much sleep can be expected was apparently very effective.

A recent report for the World Health Organization suggested that there are large differences in prescribing sleeping pills between countries. Women, particularly older women, are more likely to be prescribed sleeping pills than men (although in later life women tend to take more prescribed drugs overall than men). Unemployment, low income, bereavement, disability and long-term alcohol abuse are often found to be associated with prescribed sleeping pills. Regular night workers rely heavily on sleeping pills to help them sleep during the day, with long-term usage particularly common for this group. Yet many of these conditions suggest that physiological factors alone are unlikely to account for the prevalence of sleep disturbances or the complaints of poor sleep – in which case, pills may help in the short term, but it is equally important to tackle long-term issues.

Although it is not a good idea to rely on sleeping pills forever more, it is in fact quite common for them to be used for periods of six months or longer. After this length of time there may be withdrawal problems for certain brands, suggesting that dependency, whether physiological or psychological, is a real risk. Abuse of sleeping pills is also a concern. In Scotland, for example, one of the most commonly prescribed drugs has been used by youth cultures as a recreational drug, often in combination with other drugs. Although prescribed to aid sleep, taken in large doses this drug can have a similar uninhibiting effect to alcohol and can stimulate activity or over-excitability. This is a particularly disturbing trend, and has been linked with as many as 80 deaths in this area. In recognition of the potential social hazards, the UK have recently restricted the availability of certain sleeping pills.

Jet lag

Over the last generation or so we have seen dramatic changes in the cost and availability of world travel, with more and more people opting for exotic holiday destinations or embarking on frequent business trips around the globe. However, for many travellers the freedom to cross time zones rapidly is not without physical costs, and every day thousands of people are faced with the negative effects of trans-global travel on the body, known collectively as 'jet lag'. This description is in fact something of a misnomer, as we now know that jet lag can easily be simulated in the laboratory without even leaving the ground, or going anywhere near a plane.

In the past, it has been commonly assumed that the major problems of jet lag are something to do with the flight itself. Flights do have their own problems, particularly concerning digestion, circulation and insufficient sleep during a lengthy trip. It is also easy to become dehydrated during a trip as dry cabin air is re-circulated, a problem further exacerbated by alcohol. However, jet lag is not so much to do with the in-flight conditions of long haul flights as with the contradiction thrown up between the timing of internal body rhythms and the demands of the destination environment. As such, the problem only arises for airline passengers whose journey involves crossing time zones in a relatively short space of time. The effect of this is that the internal body clock is immediately out of synchrony with the local destination time.

The most common symptoms of jet lag include severe sleepiness or fatigue, feelings of light-headedness, nausea, dizziness, headaches, indigestion and insomnia, with obvious knock-on effects in terms of eating and social activity. These symptoms can persist for some time (on average around four to five days) as the body re-adjusts and comes in line with the new environment.

There are a number of ways of dealing with jet lag. For short trips (one to three days), it may be reasonable to continue to follow the circadian pattern familiar with home territory. This involves maintaining, as far as possible, one's original sleep and activity schedules, and ignoring the urge to follow local time. However, most people are not willing or keen to do this, as it would mean being out of step with the local events. Longer trips, whether for business or pleasure, usually necessitate a near or complete adaptation to the new time zone. It is during this adaptation period, when the body is resetting the circadian time-keepers in line with the new environment, that problems of physical discomfort can occur.

During this period, the body is exposed to the contradiction of internal and external signals. Fig 7 illustrates the demands faced during a typical journey involving a five-hour shift in time zones. This is a hypothetical westward flight (often thought to be easier on the circadian system) from London to Miami. Given a take-off time of around 11am in London, an approximately journey time of ten hours means landing in Miami at around 9pm London time. This is the time at which the body will be working towards winding down in preparation for a good night's sleep. However, because of the five-hour time difference between the cities, the time in Miami will actually be closer to 4pm on landing, and all the local activities will be geared towards late afternoon/early evening.

Thanks to the natural propensity of the circadian system towards a slightly longer than 24-hour day, it may be relatively easy to keep going on the day of travel until late into the evening. This is easier to achieve if it is possible to get out into the bright sunlight and a busy, active environment. In fact, it is a good idea to stay awake as long as possible on that first evening.

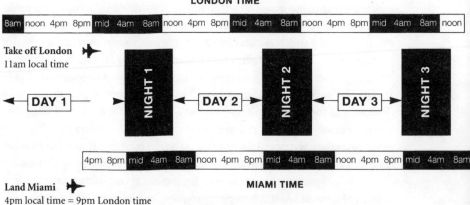

Fig 7 *A journey involving a five-hour shift in time zones.*

However, as can be seen from Fig 7, even though bedtime is likely to be much later than usual on the first night, for the next morning at least most people can expect to wake up quite a bit earlier than they might prefer. This is because the body is still literally operating on London time, even though it may be only 4am in Miami. Such an early start can lead to weariness later in the day, although long naps should be avoided, as the early-morning awakenings will gradually improve with each day and following continued exposure to the new environment. Even if you are fortunate enough to be able to lie in until 7am Miami time, as far as the body is concerned it is already noon, and this will be reflected across a range of functions, including temperature, appetite, digestion and arousal.

This confusion between internal and external influences on the body means that, for the first few days at least, we can expect to be sleepy when we would really prefer to be awake (and having fun) and wide awake in the second half of the night. Fortunately for most, within a few days the body begins to show signs of adaptation to the new environment and the effects of jet lag are gradually reduced.

There is considerable disagreement over the reasons why some people are more prone to jet lag than others. Older travellers are thought to have more difficulties but this can be hard to assess, as sleep is often problematic for the elderly. The severity of symptoms depends on how many time zones are crossed and the time difference between home and destination. On a westward flight, as in this example, adaptation is made easier, because coping with a slightly longer than normal day is within most people's capability. However, with eastward travel, day one is effectively reduced, as we arrive at a destination to find that the local time is later in the day than the starting point. A shorter day is more difficult for most people to achieve. This is described as being 'phase advanced' in relation to local time, whereas in a westward direction one is 'phase delayed'.

The powerful influence of social and environmental factors has already been discussed in relation to the 'fine-tuning' of a normal daily pattern of sleep and wake. With such an immediate transition to an unfamiliar time zone, the demands on the body to get in tune with the outside world are more dramatic. There have been many attempts to facilitate adaptation and so relieve the discomfort of jet lag. It has been suggested that during long flights, carefully timed direct exposure to bright light can be useful to reschedule the body clock in line with the destination time zone.

The development of effective techniques would no doubt be welcomed by frequent travellers or for occupations that rely on arriving at a destination feeling crisp and alert and ready for action. In anticipation of difficulties, organizations can help prepare workers before actual travel by exposing them to the alternative time schedule. For example, astronauts or military personnel can be trained to an expected shiftwork pattern to allow the crucial adaptation period to occur within the relative safety of home base and not during mission time, when it is perhaps critical for them to perform at optimum efficiency from the moment of arrival. For the military in particular, however, there may well be very little notice given before travelling, and under such circumstances it would be extremely useful to be able provide artificial 'encouragement' for the circadian system to shift without undue delay. At the moment, treatment with carefully timed exposure to bright light seems to be the most likely candidate for further development in this area.

Jet lag also takes its toll on flight crews, with studies showing the accumulated effects of ongoing sleep reduction for those working on regular long-haul flights. Airline crew may prefer to reduce the risks of jet lag by following the body's more familiar rhythm as far as possible, rather than adapting to the local environment. However, for anything longer than a one-to two-day stop-over this is likely to be extremely difficult, given the confusing distraction of natural daylight even though the body would otherwise believe it to be night. Experimental studies have highlighted the difficulties of working under conditions which place regular pressure on the circadian system, problems which may be likened to those of the more general shiftworker who is also required to make frequent adaptations to a sleep/wake schedule.

Sleep is for wimps

Accidents due to human error are far more likely to occur at certain times during the 24-hour cycle (see Chapter 12) , and it is no coincidence that these are also the times when the body's drive to sleep is at its height. Despite our best efforts, we do not perform at our best when we are tired. We are less articulate and lack the ability to interact on a social level, and this may prove crucial for certain scenarios. The *Report of the Presidential Commission on the Space Shuttle Challenger Accident* drew attention to the extensive shift hours and acute sleep deprivation of the key workers in the run-up to the crucial decision to launch[2]. This was believed to be one of the contributing factors to a breakdown in communication on certain issues. The principal author of this report was quoted as saying:

> In my opinion, fatigue is not what caused the accident, but it didn't help the decision-making process… It's another brick – the human brick.

The month before the Challenger accident, a launch accident involving the space shuttle Columbia was narrowly averted. Fuel tanks carrying liquid oxygen necessary to project the shuttle into orbit were drained inadvertently by ground crew. The operators in charge, although not aware of the major problem, did find certain related anomalies and the launch was abandoned. A report into this incident revealed that operators making critical decisions were working under demanding shift schedules (12-hour nights).

There are a number of issues here which can quickly become confused in a call for more sleep. Firstly, major slips occur when key workers are awake at a time when most people expect to be asleep. On top of this, however, there is often a degree of accumulated sleep loss, as in the run-up to an important event it is common for workers to follow long shifts and sacrifice days off as they work towards a time-critical goal. Taken together, the two factors impair performance to an extent that accidents, resulting from the oversight of important details or incapacity in dealing with complex situations, are more likely to occur.

Unfortunately, in today's society sleep is quickly abandoned at the first sign of trouble. It would be practically unheard of for a government figure to announce that they were going to bed in the middle of a crisis simply because they were tired, even though the evidence suggests that this might not be a bad idea. Instead, we hear anecdotal reports of workers staying beyond their shift and virtually 'shadowing' a replacement shift in order to keep track as a crisis develops. Consequently, the concept of crisis management often has little regard for the body's need for sleep because of the unspoken assumption that willpower alone is an adequate substitute under such conditions.

This was apparent with the NASA employees working on the space programme who, perhaps enthusiastic about the forthcoming event and undaunted by a heavy workload, should perhaps have been subject to stricter work/rest regulations. The problem in these circumstances is that work schedules are allowed to remain flexible in response to the job. In the case of space shuttle flights, for example, where delays and last-minute rescheduling are common, the sleep patterns of engineers and technicians have in the past become gradually more erratic as the final launch approaches.

In fact, many high achievers make a virtue out of going without sleep, and attribute their own successes to extended hours of productive wake, rather than 'wasting' time with sleep. Chronic short sleep is a sacrifice aspiring managers and entrepreneurs are expected to make, and this is not just at the top of the managerial profession. A recent report on British workers estimated that almost one-quarter of all full-time employed adults currently work over 50 hours per week, ie outside the recent EU directive on work hours – but at what cost in terms of productivity and restrictions on family life?

Power naps

Attitudes towards the effects of fatigue at work have taken an interesting turn over the last few years, albeit at a fairly privileged level of corporate life. Whereas sleeping during the day has long been associated with laziness and over-indulgence, a habit the modern executive has been loathe to admit to,it is now considered to be a positive boon to efficiency, thanks to its re-invention as a 'power' nap. Very short napping, sometimes as little as five to ten minutes, has been shown under experimental conditions to be an extremely effective way of relieving fatigue. It may well be that whereas caffeine and other stimulants deal with the superficial problems of sleepiness – drowsiness and fatigue – the brain is still hungry for sleep, and although more alert, the underlying cognitive problems persist. A nap, on the other hand, offers a more direct solution to controlling sleepiness and is more likely to refresh the parts caffeine cannot reach.

Often referred to as the 'Napoleonic nap' in recognition of Napoleon's disdain for extended sleep in favour of short, brief naps, the 10–15 minute power nap is considered by many to be a responsible contribution to the work environment. So convinced are some organizations of the restorative power of the nap that special areas, decorated and equipped to be conducive to sleep, are set aside for the busy executive to 'recharge' throughout the course of a long day. Not surprisingly, efficiency, even in sleep, is at a premium, with many power napping 'aids' now available, such as executive napping recliners, relaxation tapes and facial masks, all designed to speed up the transition to sleep. Whereas all the old euphemisms for afternoon sleeping ('cat napping', '40 winks', 'just resting my eyes') imply that there is something sneaky, mischievous or time-wasting about this habit, the 'power nap' on the other hand describes time well spent in restoring the individual to their more formidable alert self.

So if sleep has been at least partially revamped as a more acceptable activity, who is power napping? As you might expect, this is the prerogative of the 'decision-makers' higher up the chain of command, while sleeping on the job is still actively discouraged in most other areas of the workplace.

The specifics of qualitative aspects of napping are still debatable, although some people claim that switching off for a just a few minutes can have a positive effect. There are potential drawbacks to sleeping during the day, though. It is important to avoid what starts out as a 'nap' developing into a more profound sleep (ie longer than about 20 minutes), as the grogginess which follows can be difficult to shake off. Long naps during the day can also impinge on the need for sleep at night, making it difficult to sleep at the normal time or for as long as we might like.

But again, this is not predictable. One of the reasons for this is that we cannot always distinguish between sleep that we genuinely need and sleeping for reasons which have more to do with the environment or state of mind. We sometimes nap for sheer pleasure, or so it seems, although current thinking assumes that napping, although often pleasurable, serves a more essential purpose. In one form or another, the daytime nap seems to have re-emerged as a regular feature of many people's pattern of sleep and it had been argued that this is indicative of a more sinister, underlying sleep debt. Certainly, the ability to nap is in direct relation to how well we have slept at night, with more people nowadays admitting either that they are sleeping during the day, or that they would very much like the opportunity.

What is 'normal'?

Data from surveys carried out recently suggest that most people endorse a 'common-sense' belief that we need eight hours' sleep each night. There is no such thing as the 'average' sleeper, however. All the signs indicate a wide range of sleep needs across the general population (see Part 2), with some people managing quite well on four hours and others determined that they need much closer to nine or even ten hours each night. It has not been possible to discover what it is about individual constitutions that makes this so – neither personality nor physiology provides a simple explanation. Life circumstances are an important factor and, within limits, we all seem to have a degree of flexibility in our sleep patterns to enable us to cope will sudden changes in sleep brought about by circumstance or necessity.

Today, we are also relatively unique in organizing sleep and activity patterns around a complex series of social activities. Consequently, we are faced with a daily competition between socially determined work and leisure patterns and physiological processes representing an intrinsic need for sleep. Our decision to sleep is often a compromise between these competing factors. So, from time to time when these predictable and habit-driven 'zeitgebers' are loosened, we are able to re-adjust our sleep patterns to a limited extent to suit the current situation. On holidays or at weekends, for example, when there is no longer an incentive to get up for work, we may choose to stay in bed for an hour or so longer. During experimental confinement, when volunteers are limited in what they are able to do by way of amusement or distraction and are presented with few alternatives to sleep, there is a tendency for them to doze lightly whenever they can, and at all hours of the day if possible. Under these circumstances, people are highly motivated to sleep simply because they are bored.

There is often the paradoxical finding that, given the opportunity to sleep longer than normal, people actually feel less refreshed than on their routine 'shorter' night of sleep. The reasons for this are unclear, and by no means everybody develops these complaints, but feeling groggy or fatigued after a lie in can give the impression that even more sleep is needed. In these circumstances, however, sleeping on is often counterproductive, and the only real remedy is to get up and be active.

The perception of having had enough sleep often has little to do with how long we have slept for. People who describe themselves as 'poor sleepers' may actually sleep for quite substantial amounts of time, but are disturbed by the quality of sleep, which is usually shallower or more frequently interrupted than for others. Feeling refreshed in the morning and having the sense of having slept well depends on many factors, not simply how long we have slept. There is therefore no guarantee that by allotting 'sufficient' time for sleep we will necessarily fill this with 'quality' sleep.

Towards a world without sleep?

The claim that we are sleeping less than previous generations is often made in relation to a limited amount of data concerning sleep habits around the turn of the century. Yet evidence for change is slim, with considerable contradiction between historical studies. Even so, the possibility that we are sleeping less has intuitive appeal in view of the fact that the world is described as a more complex place. Perhaps more importantly, though, we should be concerned as to whether the extent of this presumed reduction in sleep (usually estimated at between 30 and 90 minutes per night) and its placement throughout the day/night period is outside a more general human sleep need.

What seems to have happened over the past century is that we are now sleeping 'differently'. Contemporary work and social environments are not only more complex, but also more artificial in terms of light/dark and quiet/active cycles. Whereas activity might once have been determined by the natural availability of light, this distinction has now been flattened out, with the effect that we rely more heavily on socially determined influences to discipline the internal rhythms of the body than ever before. The challenge for the future is to identify risk areas outside the limits of human flexibility. Under controlled conditions, for example, it has been possible to show that a gradual reduction of sleep is well tolerated, but that we are not so good at making abrupt changes. But these conditions rarely take into account the additional pressures and demands likely to necessitate less sleep, or the rather dismissive assumption that sleep is an unnecessary and perhaps outmoded distraction characterized by the 'life is not a dress rehearsal' approach. For many people, the possibility of alternatives to sleep is an attractive one, although available alternatives make poor substitutes in the long run.

Finally, thanks to recent technological developments we are closer than ever to describing the mechanics of the sleep process. We are also more competent in measuring actual sleep in the population, and highlighting the existence of problem areas. The ability to describe sleep in greater detail and with more precision has coincided with a broadening of interest in this behaviour to include not only medical and scientific but also many educational, legal and social concerns. As such, a responsible attitude towards sleep is currently considered to be vital for personal achievement and individual social responsibility.

The aim of this book has been to consider the development of interest and research into sleep, in line with developments in all areas of modern life. At times it has been a selective account, although not with the intention of promoting a particular point of view. Rather, it has tried to show that sleep is a multi-faceted subject – attracting many different perspectives and approaches, and seeming to generate as many questions as answers.

References

The material covered in this book has been selected from a wide range of sources. The following references provide suggestions for further reading and cover a mixture of popular books, available from good bookshops, and journal reports, more likely to be found in the local university library. Most of the older experimental reports, in particular, are well known and likely to be covered in modern texts. In addition, the Internet now provides access to good quality information and discussion across a range of sleep-related issues, with many university or medical sites offering a useful starting point for investigation.

Part 1

Chapter 1
1 Robinson, E.S., & Richardson-Robinson, F. 'Effects of loss of sleep', *Journal of Experimental Psychology*, Vol 15, pp93–100 (1922).
2 Kleitman, N. *Sleep and Wakefulness* (Chicago University Press, 1963).
3 Lewis, P.R., & Lobban, M.C. 'Dissociation of diurnal rhythms in human subjects living on abnormal time routines', *Quarterly Journal of Experimental Physiology*, Vol 42, pp371–86 (1957) .

Chapter 2
1 Frazer, J. *The Golden Bough* (1922). The Wordsworth Reference edition provides an abridged version of an earlier work and includes a fascinating account of the way sleep and dreaming was viewed as central to community life for primitive cultures.
See also:
Lincoln, J.S. *The Dream in Primitive Cultures* (The Cressett Press, London, 1935).
Megroz, R.L. *The Dream World: A Survey of the History and Mystery of Dreams* (The Bodley Head, London, 1939).

2 Howell, J. *British or Old Cambrian Proverbs* (1659).
3 Scot, R. *The Discoverie of Witchcraft* (1584).
4 Ray, J. *A Collection of English Proverbs* (1670).

Part 2

Chapter 4
1 Wilcox, R.H. 'Awakening as an operant behaviour: preliminary results', *Physiology and Behaviour*, Vol 14, pp345–51 (1975).
2 Oosterhuis, A., & Klip, E.C. 'The treatment of insomnia through mass media, the results of a televised behavioural training programme', *Social Science and Medicine*, Vol 45(8), pp1223–9 (1997)
3 Kageyama, T., Kabuto, M., Nitta, N., et al. 'A cross-sectional study on insomnia among Japanese adult women in relation to night-time road traffic noise', *Journal of Sound and Vibration*, Vol 205(4), pp387–91 (1997).
4 Hofman, W.F., Kumar, A., & Tulen, J.H.M. 'Cardiac reactivity to traffic noise during sleep in man', *Journal of Sound and Vibration*, Vol 179(4), pp577–89 (1995).
5 Partinen, M., Putkonen, P.T.S., Kaprio, J., & Kosvenvuo, M. 'Genetic and environmental

determination of human sleep', *Sleep*, Vol 6(3), pp179–85 (1983).
6 Palmer, C.D., Harrison, G.A., & Hiorns, R.W. 'Association between smoking and drinking and sleep duration', *Annals of Human Biology*, Vol 7(2), pp103–7 (1980).

Chapter 5
1 Kripke, D.F., Simons, R.N., Garfinkel. M.A., & Hammond, E.C. 'Short and long sleep and sleeping pills', *Archives of General Psychiatry*, Vol 36, pp103–16 (1979).
2 Belloc, N.B., & Breslow, L. 'Relationship of physical health status and health practices', *Preventive Medicine*, Vol 1, pp409–21 (1972) / Wingard, D.L., & Berkman, L.F. 'Mortality risk associated with sleeping patterns among adults', *Sleep*, Vol 6(2), pp102–7 (1983).
3 Hulshof, K.F.A.M., Wedel, M., Lowik, M.R.H., et al. 'Clustering of dietary variables and other lifestyle factors (Dutch Nutritional Surveillance System)', *Journal of Epidemiology and Community Health*, Vol 46, pp417–24 (1992).
4 Mattiasson, I., Lindgarde, F., Nilsson, J.A., & Theorell, T. 'Threat of unemployment and cardiovascular risk factors: longitudinal study of quality of sleep and serum choles-terol concentrations in men threatened with redundancy', *British Medical Journal*, Vol 301, pp461–6 (1990).
5 Hyyppa, M.T., Kronholm, E., & Alanen, E. 'Quality of sleep during economic recession in Finland: a longitudinal cohort study', *Social Science and Medicine*, Vol 45(5), pp731–8 (1997).
6 Ferrie, J.E., Shipley, M.J., Marmot, M.G., et al. 'The health effects of major organi-zational change and job insecurity', *Social Science and Medicine*, Vol 46(2), pp243–54 (1998).
7 Raggatt, P.T.F. 'Work stress among long-distance coach drivers: a survey and correlational study', *Journal of Organizational Behaviour*, Vol 12, pp565–79 (1991).
8 Guerrero, J., & Crocq, M. 'Sleep disorders in the elderly: depression and post-traumatic stress disorder', *Journal of Psychosomatic Research*, Vol 38, suppl 1, pp141–50 (1994).

Chapter 7
1 Baildam, E.M., Hillier, V.F., Ward, B.S., Bannister, R.P., Bamford, F.N., Moore, W.M.O. 'Duration and pattern of crying in the first year of life', *Developmental Medicine and Child Neurology*, Vol 37, pp345–53 (1995).
2 Gau, S.F., & Soong, W.T. 'Sleep problems of junior high school students in Tapei', *Sleep*, Vol 18(8), pp667–73 (1995).
3 Terman, L.M., & Hocking, A. 'The sleep of school children: its distribution according to age, and its relation to physical and mental efficiency', *Journal of Educational Psychology*, Vol 4, pp138–289 (1913).
4 Weissbluth, M., Poncher, J., Given, G., et al. 'Sleep duration and television viewing', *The Journal of Pediatrics*, Vol 99(3), pp486–8 (1981).

Chapter 8
1 These cases were reported in the *Daily Telegraph* (Saturday 12 October 1996). Although there are very few accounts of such cases of 'total' chronic insomnia, medial textbooks may provide further information.

Part 3

Chapter 9
1 Freud, S. *On Dreams* (William Heineman (Medical Books) Ltd, London, 1914).
Or, for a more modern account :
Welsh, A. *Freud's Wishful Dream Book* (Princeton University Press, Princeton, NJ, 1994).
For earlier ideas on sleep and dreaming, see also:
Hine, R. L. *Dreams and the Way of Dreams* (J.M. Dent & Sons Ltd, London, 1913).
Valentine, C.W. *Dreams and the Unconscious* (Christophers, London, 1921).
Rivers, W.H.R. 'Freud's psychology of the unconscious', *The Lancet*, pp912–14 (16 June 1917).
2 Aserinsky, E., & Kleitman, N. 'Two types of ocular motility occurring in sleep', *Journal of Applied Physiology*, Vol 8, pp1–10 (1955).
3 *See for example:* Dement, W.C., & Fisher, C. 'Experimental interference with the sleep cycle', *Canadian Psychiatric Association*

Journal, Vol 8 (6), pp400–5 (1993)/Dement, W. 'The effect of dream deprivation', *Science,* Vol 131(3415), pp1705–7 (1960).

Chapter 10
1 Barker, J.C. 'Premonitions of the Aberfan disaster', *Journal of the Society for Psychical Research,* Vol 44(734), pp169–81 (1967). Barker also went on the establish the British Premonitions Bureau.
2 Dunne, J.W. *An Experiment with Time* (Faber, 1927).
3 Besterman, T. 'Report of inquiry into precognitive dreams', *Journal of the Society for Psychical Research,* Vol 41, pp186–204 (1933).
4 Lewicki, D.R., Schaut, G.H., & Persinger, M.A. 'Geophysical variables and behaviour: XLIV. Days of subjective precognitive experiences and the days before the actual events display correlated geomagnetic activity', *Perceptual and Motor Skills,* Vol 65, pp173–4 (1986).
5 Cox, W.E. 'Precognition: An analysis. II', *Journal of the American Society for Psychical Research,* Vol 50, pp99–109 (1956).

Chapter 11
1 Twemlow, S.W., Baggard, G.O., & Jones, F.C. 'The out-of-body experience: a phenomenological typology based on questionnaire responses', *American Journal of Psychiatry,* Vol 139 (4), pp450–5 (1982).
2 Sheils, D. 'A cross-cultural study of beliefs in out-of-body experiences, waking and sleeping', *Journal of the Society for Psychical Research,* Vol 49(755), pp697–741 (1978).
See also:
Hadfield, J.A. *Dreams and Nightmares* (Penguin Books, Middlesex, 1954).
Mavromatis, A. *Hypnagogia: The Unique State of Consciousness Between Wakefulness and Sleep* (Routledge & Kegan Paul, London & New York, 1987).

Part 4

Chapter 12
1 Irwin, H.J. 'The psychological function of out-of-body experiences: so who needs the out-of-body experience?', *The Journal of* *Nervous and Mental Disease,* Vol 169(4), pp244–8 (1981)/Sheils, D. 'A cross-cultural study of beliefs in out-of-body experiences, waking and sleeping', *Journal of the Society for Psychical Research,* Vol 49(755), pp697–741 (1978).

Chapter 13
1 Mitler, M.M., Carskadon, M.A., Czeisler, C.A., et al. 'Catastrophes, sleep, and public policy: a consensus report', *Sleep,* Vol 11(1), 100–9 (1988).
2 *Report of the Presidential Commission on the Space Shuttle Challenger Accident.* Hearings were held between 26 February and 2 May 1986. Press reports around this time also give summary reports of the Commission's main findings.
3 Bjerner, B., Holm, A., & Swensson, A. 'Diurnal variation in mental performance', *British Journal of Industrial Medicine,* Vol 12, pp103–10 (1955).
4 Leger, D. 'The cost of sleep-related accidents – a report for the National Commission on Sleep Disorders Research', *Sleep,* Vol 17(1), pp84–93 (1994).
5 Kay v Butterworth, *Justice of the Peace and Local Government Review Reports,* Vol 75, p110 (1946).
6 Brown, I. D., Tickner, A.H., & Simmonds, D.C.V. 'Effect of prolonged driving on over-taking criteria', *Ergonomics,* Vol 13(2), 239–42 (1970).
7 There are also many sources of discussion and debate concerning this report on the Internet.
8 These issues were discussed in a series of articles published in the medical and popular press, including: Asch, D.A., & Parker, R.M. 'The Libby Zion case – one step forward or two steps backward?', *The New England Medical Journal,* Vol 318(12), pp771–5 (1988).
9 'The dangers of not going to bed', *The Lancet* (21 January 1989). Editorial on junior hospital doctors' work hours.

Chapter 14
1 The case of Parks is reported in the *Canadian Law Reports* (R v Parks (1992) 75 CCC (3d)), although will no doubt be included in future discussions in popular texts.

2–4 *For a discussion of the earliest cases see:* Walker, N. *Crime and Insanity in England, Vol 1: The Historical Perspective,* pp165–77 (The University Press, Edinburgh, 1968).

5 Although not reported in the *Law Journals,* this case has been described elsewhere, including: Howard, C., & D'Orban, P.T., 'Violence in sleep: medicolegal issues and two case reports', *Psychological Medicine,* Vol 17, pp915–25 (1987).

6 *See* Walker, (2–4) above.

7 *See* Howard & D'Orban, (5) above.

8 The case of Boshears was covered in the media but not in the *Law Reports. See: The Times* (3 January and 17–18 February 1961).

9 Tarsh, M.J. 'On serious violence during sleep-walking' (letter), *British Journal of Psychiatry,* Vol 148, p476 (1986).

10 *See* Howard & D'Orban, (5) above/Oswald, I., & Evans, J. 'On serious violence during sleep-walking', *British Journal of Psychiatry,* Vol 147, pp688–91 (1985).

11 The case involving Kemp was widely reported at the time, including: *The Times* (3 May 1986)/ Schatzman, M., 'To sleep, perchance to kill', *The New Scientist,* Vol 110(1514), pp60–2 (1986).

12 R v Burgess (2 QB 92 at 99, 1991).

13 Nofzinger, E.A., & Wettstein, R.M. 'Homicidal behaviour and sleep apnoea: a case report and medico-legal discussion', *Sleep,* Vol 18(9), pp776–82 (1995).

14 Bratty v A-G (Northern Ireland AC 386, 1963). Also to be found in discussions outside the law reports.

15 Roper, P. 'Bulimia while sleep-walking, a rebuttal for sane automatism?', *The Lancet,* p796 (30 September 1989).

For an interesting and up-to-date review of this area, see also: Thomas, T.N. 'Sleepwalking disorder and Mens Rea: a review and case report', *Journal of Forensic Science,* Vol 42(1), pp17–24 (1997).

Chapter 15

1 Hawkins, J., & Shaw, P. 'Sleep satisfaction and intentional self-awakening: an alternative protocol for self-report data', *Perceptual and Motor Skills,* Vol 70, pp447–50 (1990).

2 *Report of the Presidential Commission on the Space Shuttle Challenger Accident – see above (Chapter 13).*

Index

Page numbers in *italics* refer to the figures and tables